MELATONIN

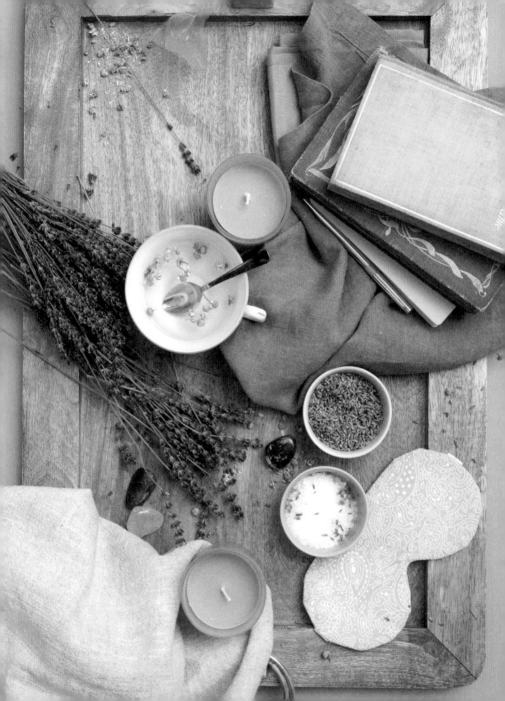

RITUAL WELLNESS

MELATONIN

The Natural Supplement for Better Sleep

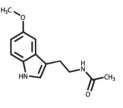

Locke Hughes

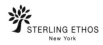

STERLING ETHOS
New York

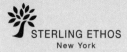

STERLING ETHOS
New York

An Imprint of Sterling Publishing Co., Inc.
1166 Avenue of the Americas
New York, NY 10036

This publication includes alternative therapies that have not been scientifically tested, is intended for
informational purposes only, and is not intended to provide or replace conventional medical advice,
treatment or diagnosis or be a substitute to consulting with licensed medical or health-care providers.
The publisher does not claim or guarantee any benefits, healing, cure or any results in any respect and
shall not be liable or responsible for any use or application of any content in this publication in any respect
including without limitation any adverse effects, consequence, loss or damage of any type resulting or
arising from, directly or indirectly, any use or application of any content herein. Any trademarks are the
property of their respective owners, are used for editorial purposes only, and the publisher makes no claim
of ownership and shall acquire no right, title or interest in such trademarks by virtue of this publication.

ISBN 978-1-4549-3766-1

Distributed in Canada by Sterling Publishing Co., Inc.
c/o Canadian Manda Group, 664 Annette Street
Toronto, Ontario M6S 2C8, Canada
Distributed in the United Kingdom by GMC Distribution Services
Castle Place, 166 High Street, Lewes, East Sussex BN7 1XU, England
Distributed in Australia by NewSouth Books
University of New South Wales, Sydney, NSW 2052, Australia

For information about custom editions, special sales, and premium and corporate
purchases, please contact Sterling Special Sales at 800-805-5489 or
specialsales@sterlingpublishing.com.

Manufactured in Canada

2 4 6 8 10 9 7 5 3 1

sterlingpublishing.com

Cover design by David Ter-Avanesyan
Cover photography by Christopher Bain
Cover image of molecule by Leonid Andronov/Shutterstock.com
Interior design by Ashley Prine, Tandem Books

For picture credits, see page 143

"O sleep, O gentle sleep.
I thought gratefully,
Nature's gentle nurse!"

—Elizabeth Kenny,
Australian nurse and health
administrator (1880–1952)

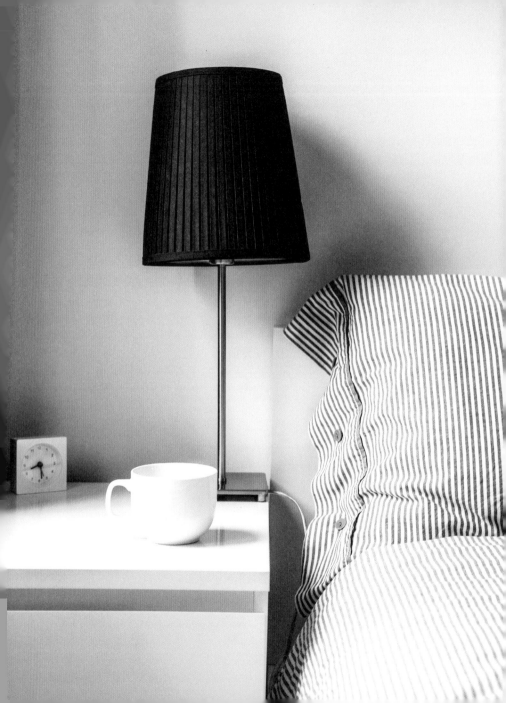

CONTENTS

INTRODUCTION

Let's start with a simple question: How'd you sleep last night? I'll venture a guess that you probably mumbled "fine" in response, shrugged your shoulders, and took yet another sip of coffee. But I bet that sleeping "fine" isn't cutting it—not for your health, productivity, or relationships.

Perhaps "fine" means that you got a decent night's sleep—seven hours or so—with a few wake-ups or bathroom visits along the way. Actually, come to think of it, it was probably more like five or six hours.

Or maybe you got in bed early, but after a few minutes of tossing and turning, you reached for your phone and started scrolling through social media and video clips until the early morning hours. Or perhaps you've been traveling across multiple time zones, which can make it nearly impossible to fall asleep at an appropriate time, no matter how tired you might feel. Whatever your typical nighttime routine looks like, it's probably not *really* "fine," is it? After all, you did pick up this book.

I can relate. I too have experienced years of frustrating, fragmented, and fitful nights of sleep. In those days, I felt irritable, anxious, and distracted—just a few of the inevitable side effects of sleeplessness. Every day, around 3 p.m., whether I was at my desk or at home, a sense of heaviness and fatigue would set in, and it was all I could do to keep my eyes open. Sometimes, I didn't. (My apologies to my coworkers; it wasn't you—it was me.) I began to feel hopeless and burned out; I'd lost the energy to do things that brought me joy.

Put simply, I was exhausted—and it affected my entire life. But, like you, I was far from alone. Most people around the world aren't getting enough sleep. In fact, two out of three adults in all developed nations don't obtain the recommended eight hours of sleep per night, and our collective inability to catch sufficient shut-eye has become such an issue for our health and well-being that the World Health Organization (WHO) has declared a sleep-loss "epidemic."

What's more, countries where the average time people sleep has declined most dramatically over the past century—including the US, the UK, Japan, South Korea, and several countries in western Europe—have also witnessed an increase in rates of physical disease and mental disorders as a result of insufficient sleep. Forget our common humanity, it's sleep deficiency that seems to be the international currency that unites us around the world. While the causes may be varied and complex, we all simply want to *sleep*.

The good news? We can.

It is possible to get a good night's rest, without resorting to expensive medications that knock you out into oblivion. It is possible to feel rested and alert, not weary and drowsy, when you wake up in the morning.

It's all possible, thanks to melatonin, a hormone that our bodies create naturally. We just have to learn how to harness its power, nurture its production, and if necessary, how to supplement it.

In the following pages, I'll introduce you to the melatonin your body produces as well as the supplement. I'll elucidate how both can help you fall asleep and bestow numerous other health benefits.

But there's a catch. (There's always a catch!) Melatonin alone isn't enough to improve your sleep (nor your life) permanently. That's why this book will also cover the importance of sleep hygiene as well as bedtime routines and how to figure out which one works best for you. Finally, you'll find delicious recipes that are simple to make—and that can help deliver you to dreamland, quickly and calmly.

The information in this book has the potential to change your life— just as it has changed mine. Today, I no longer find myself dozing off or losing concentration every afternoon. I don't dread the sound of my alarm in the morning. I've lost the weight I could never shake, transformed my relationships, and skyrocketed to success in my career. All thanks to knowing the secrets of sleep—and the hormone that controls it.

If you too would like to feel more energized, healthier, and happier— every day, and all day—keep reading. This book will show you how.

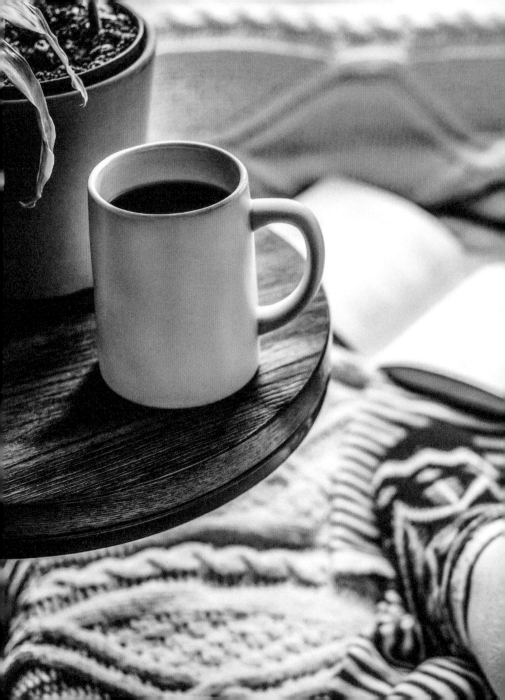

CHAPTER ONE

The Exhaustion Epidemic

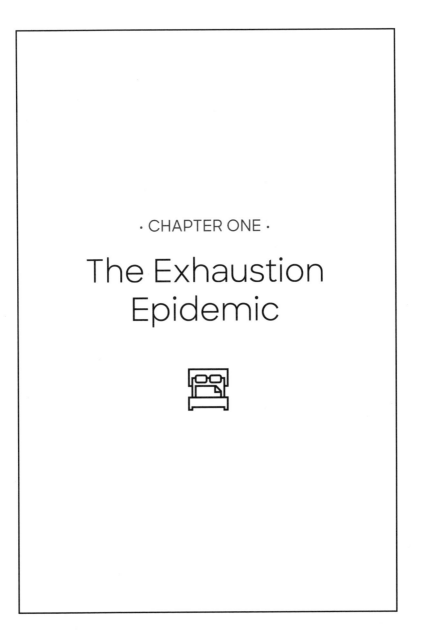

People all over the world suffer from poor sleep—regardless of country, class, or career path. The majority of people (notably, 56 percent in the US and Japan, and 66 percent in Germany) say they don't catch enough zzz's during the week, according to a 2013 poll conducted by the National Sleep Foundation.

The same survey also asked participants how often they can say that they had "a good night's sleep." In the UK, 11 percent of people said they can *never* say that. In the US, 20 percent of people said they *rarely* can, as did 17 percent of people in Canada. Seventy-six percent of Americans reported feeling tired at work many days of the week, while 23 percent said they had problems concentrating during the day due to poor sleep. In fact, with more than 70 million American adults suffering from a sleep disorder, the Centers for Disease Control and Prevention (CDC) has declared insufficient sleep to be a public health epidemic.

And it's not just industrialized nations suffering from sleep issues. In a large-scale survey of more than 18,000 people from 134 countries known as The Rest Test, a shocking 68 percent of people say that they would like to get more rest. That means that most of us—7 out of 10—are living our lives exhausted.

What's more, an analysis of more than 40,000 adults across developing nations in Africa and Asia also found that an estimated 150 million people were suffering from sleep-related problems. This equals a rate of about 17 percent of the population reporting insomnia and other severe sleep disturbances—nearly the 20 percent found in the general adult population in the West.

The thing is, we haven't always been so sleep deprived. In 1942, Americans were sleeping an average of 7.9 hours per night, but by 2013, that had dropped to 6.8 hours per night—below the recommended minimum of seven hours for optimal health and well-being. If we used to get more sleep in the past, what's changed?

SLEEP HABITS THROUGHOUT HISTORY

The Neolithic Era (began around 10,000 BCE): Our ancestors likely went to sleep on piles of hay shortly after the sun set to reduce the dangers posed by nocturnal predators.

The Renaissance (1300-1600): During this time of social and artistic advancements, a biphasic sleep pattern—meaning two separate periods of sleep—was common. People would have a "first sleep" about two hours after dusk. Then they'd wake up for one or two hours, during which time they might pray, reflect, have sex, complete chores, or read by candlelight. Then they'd have a "second sleep" for another four hours or so until morning.

The Industrial Revolution (1760-1840): As people started to work long days in factories, biphasic sleep faded out in favor of a single sleep cycle of about eight hours.

Modern Day (1840-present): The invention of the electric lightbulb in the late nineteenth century has vastly impacted our sleep schedules. With more exposure to light late in the evening, we delay the signal from our internal clock telling us it's time to sleep. (Read more on how light impacts our sleep in chapter 2.)

WHY ARE WE SO TIRED?

In order to understand why we're not sleeping enough, let's begin by talking about everything we do—*besides* sleep.

Modern society seems to stimulate us to work more, play more, and socialize more—essentially, do anything *but* sleep. We wake up, check our email, grab a cup of coffee, rush to the gym (maybe), rush to the office, rush to meetings, and squeeze in social plans or family obligations after work. Then we spend our evenings glued to TV, computer, or phone screens until we finally doze off to dreamland (if we're lucky).

Today, the lines between work and personal time are blurring. Scratch that, they've already blurred beyond recognition. Thanks to our smartphones, being "on call" is no longer reserved just for doctors— we're *all* always on call. Our screens are usually the first thing we see in the morning and the last thing we see before we go to sleep. Because of the blue light waves they emit, sleeping with our screens is a serious obstacle, as we'll discuss in chapter 2.

We also struggle with our personal sleep demons, whether it's our sleeping environment or the stage of life we're in. Sleep hygiene (the act of controlling your environment in order to optimize sleep) comes up in more detail in chapter 4, but just a heads up: You're probably "trying to sleep" all wrong. We're never taught "how to sleep" in school. And if we bring it up to our doctors, they usually aren't much help in this area. Research has found that most physicians receive less than two hours of training about the entire field of sleep in their four years of medical education, and that the subject of sleep is woefully underrepresented in medical textbooks.

Surveys also show that more than 60 percent of adults have never been asked about the quality of their sleep by a physician. Fewer than

20 percent have ever initiated such a discussion—despite the fact that it's one of the most common problems that patients want to address.

All in all, it seems that being busy has become a badge of honor and rest has fallen by the wayside. In the 1800s, the upper class prided themselves on how much leisure time they had. Today, the opposite is true. It's the number of hours we work—not the amount of downtime we enjoy—that bestows social status, respect, and success.

But there are clear signs that being busy isn't working out as well as we may think. Consider that a whole new "wellness" industry dedicated to helping people relax has sprung up—from phone-free, digital detox "camps" for adults to meditation studios opening up in cities across the country.

Although we typically have a full sixteen hours each day to "get it all done" (that sounds like a good bit of time, doesn't it?), it seems we still find ourselves overbooked, overscheduled, and overwhelmed. And as our work, family, and social obligations (and worries) seep into the eight hours that used to be reserved for sleep, the effects are far more harmful than you might imagine.

THE POWER OF SLEEP

At this point, you may still be wondering whether or not insufficient sleep truly needs to be considered a "public health epidemic." You may think that sounds a bit excessive. You may feel as though a lack of sleep isn't nearly as bad as smoking cigarettes, taking drugs, or drinking too much alcohol. You're just a little tired, that's all.

That thought process does not give sleep its proper due. Sleep plays a starring role in our physical and mental health—and, in effect, our entire lives. Sleep is one of the primary human drives we need to fulfill in order to survive, along with the instincts to eat, drink water, and reproduce. While the purpose of sleep may not be as obvious as why we need to eat or reproduce, for instance, the consequences of ignoring it aren't very nice. After all, we sleep away about one-third of our lives—and during that time we can't eat, hunt, learn, work, or reproduce. So, sleep must serve *some* evolutionary purpose, right?

Indeed it does. While scientists have been studying sleep for millennia, there's not a single answer to the question of why humans sleep in the first place, although multiple theories have been posed. One of the earliest theories is the adaptive, or evolutionary, theory, which posits that lying still at night during sleep was a survival strategy to avoid predators. This was later disproven as staying aware of our surroundings is a safer strategy for avoiding danger.

Another theory suggests that sleep helps to restore our brain's energy, since the sleeping brain uses only half the amount of glucose (essentially fuel) as it does when awake. There is also a theory that sleep allows the brain to clear out toxins and "cleanse" itself, while yet another theory says sleep plays a major role in the brain's ability to learn, store memories, pay attention, and regulate emotions.

Turns out, the question of why we sleep doesn't have just one simple answer. As Matthew Walker, PhD, writes in *Why We Sleep*, "We sleep for a rich litany of functions, plural—an abundant constellation of nighttime benefits that service both our brains and our bodies."

Sleep benefits every single organ in our body, as well as every process within our brain. In order to understand what sleep does for our health, the next few sections will elucidate how a lack of sleep affects our body and mind. You'll probably be surprised at how far-reaching—and how harmful—the effects of sleep deprivation can be. As W. Chris Winter, board-certified sleep-medicine specialist, puts it in his book, *The Sleep Solution*, "Long-term poor sleep is like bad cosmetic surgery: risky, costly, and not pretty."

Sleep and Your Physical Health

Let's start on an individual level. To put it simply (and starkly), people who don't get enough sleep are at higher risk for a range of medical conditions—including obesity, diabetes, depression, hypertension, heart disease, and neurodegenerative disorders like Alzheimer's.

Our brains seem to be the organ most impacted by sleep. Researchers have found it plays a key role in helping promote brain "plasticity," or the brain's ability to change and reorganize itself. Plus, decades of sleep research have shown that sleep is largely a "brain-focused phenomenon," which explains why a lack of sleep is linked to cognitive diseases like Alzheimer's.

That's not to say sleep doesn't affect many other parts of our bodies. If you routinely sleep less than seven hours a night, it can weaken your immune system. The quality of your sleep can predict whether you catch a cold and how severe it is. Some studies suggest that those who get six hours or less of sleep have 50 percent less immunity protection than those who get eight hours per night.

This doesn't make you more likely to just catch a cold; it also more than doubles your risk of cancer. Emerging research has found a strong link between poor sleep and breast cancer, which encouraged the WHO to classify shift work as a "probable" (or class 2A) carcinogen.

If you sleep poorly, other consequences include an unhealthy heart and a shorter life span. A 2011 study looked at more than half a million men and women across nine countries and found shorter sleep durations were associated with a 45 percent increased risk of developing and/or dying of coronary heart disease within seven to twenty-five years from the start of the study.

A similar relationship was observed in a Japanese study of over four thousand male workers. Those sleeping six hours or less were 400 to 500 percent more likely to suffer one or more cardiac arrests than those sleeping more than six hours. Countless other studies have shown that a lack of shut-eye leads to an increased risk for heart attack, elevated blood pressure, heart failure, and stroke.

Sleep and Your Mental Health

It's not just your physical heart that's at risk; your heartfelt emotions are also affected by poor sleep. Lack of sleep intensifies our negative moods, such as anger, hostility, depression, confusion, tension, and sadness, while reducing our positive moods, including alertness and happiness. That means your lack of sleep—and resulting grumpy attitude—may have an unfortunate side effect on your relationships, both at home and at work.

Beyond a bad mood, poor sleep is also associated with chronic mental health problems, including depression and anxiety. In fact, difficulty sleeping is one of the main criteria that mental health professionals use to diagnose depression—that's how inextricably linked depression is with sleep problems.

Fatigue also has a range of side effects on your work performance. It's been proven to impair our cognitive capacity, reduce creativity, decrease learning ability and problem solving, impact memory, and lower motivation. Not exactly the formula to get a promotion—or even to keep a steady job.

Sleep and Your Appearance

Sleeping Beauty was clearly onto something. Besides all the internal consequences, a lack of sleep also has plenty of more noticeable complications. (Though a bad mood can certainly be obvious at times!)

As you sleep, your skin produces collagen, which is a protein that helps make your skin strong, plump, and less likely to wrinkle. Blood flow to the skin is also boosted while you snooze, giving you that healthy glow when you get enough sleep—and a drab, dull complexion if you skimp.

Chances are you've noticed dark circles around your eyes when you don't get enough sleep. This occurs because the blood in our faces isn't flowing as well when we're tired, so it can pool under our eyes. The thin skin in that area can make this even more apparent. Puffiness around the eyes is another side effect of too little shut-eye, again because the blood isn't flowing as well as it should.

A lack of sleep can also make us more likely to gain weight, since it affects the hunger hormones ghrelin and leptin. The less sleep we get, the more ghrelin (the hormone that makes us hungry) is produced, while levels of leptin (the hormone that signals us to stop eating) are reduced. That's why you feel like eating more on days after a restless night's sleep.

As a double whammy, when you're tired, your body's hunger signals are urging you to eat higher-calorie foods—hence the reason bagels, chips, and fries look so appealing when you're worn out. That's why long-term sleep deficiency will probably cause you to pack on a few pounds. In fact, a 2015 study showed that when people went to bed one hour later than usual, they gained 2.1 points on their body mass index over time.

SLEEP IN SOCIETY

On a final (and scary) note, sleep deprivation can lead to deadly consequences in a much more immediate way. Feeling sleepy affects not only your reaction time, but also your ability to pay attention and make smart decisions. When people are tired, we're much more prone to making blunders, such as fatal car accidents or medical mistakes.

Between 2005 and 2009 there was an estimated average of 83,000 crashes each year related to drowsy driving—886 of which were fatal. (Yikes!) Research from the CDC has also found that about one in twenty-five American adults admit to having fallen asleep at the wheel in the previous thirty days. (Double yikes!)

As if that's not scary enough, the doctors who are supposedly there to help may be making matters worse. Physicians, especially resident physicians, are notorious for working insanely long hours. In America, residents work a whopping eighty hours per week (which is especially rough compared to the UK's fifty-hour limit) and that's on top of sleepless nights spent on call.

This can have fatal consequences. One study reported that sleep-deprived surgeons made 20 percent more errors and took 14 percent longer to complete tasks than those who had a full night's sleep. And obviously, mistakes in the medical field shouldn't be taken lightly. A report from the Institute of Medicine revealed that medical errors cause between 44,000 and 98,000 deaths a year.

Still convinced that poor sleep isn't that bad? Consider this: Sleep deprivation is literally torture. Sleep deprivation was first documented as a way to punish prisoners in the fifteenth century. Since then, terrorists and intelligence agents alike have denied sleep to people in an attempt to elicit intel. It was an especially favored tactic of the KGB and the Japanese during World War II.

SOME GOOD NEWS

After that downer of a section, here's a positive news flash: Your sleep deficiency *can* be reversed. Although it won't happen overnight (pun intended), you *can* catch up on sleep, repay your sleep debt, and improve your health by learning the best practices for better zzz's.

While not getting enough sleep is bad, getting *good* sleep can be truly life changing. Below are the major benefits that good sleep can have on your health:

- It helps your brain store memories, cement new memories and recently learned skills, and even work out logical decisions.
- It's crucial for your heart health and your cardiovascular system, and it helps lower blood pressure.
- It helps to recalibrate and balance your emotional health.
- It restores your immune system, helping prevent illness and infection.
- It helps to fine-tune the balance of insulin and glucose.
- It regulates your appetite and controls your body weight.

In sum, as author and coach Brad Stulberg puts it, "If you could bottle up sleep and sell it as a performance-enhancing drug it would be a billion-dollar blockbuster." Melatonin might just be the next best thing—and I'll show you why, coming up next.

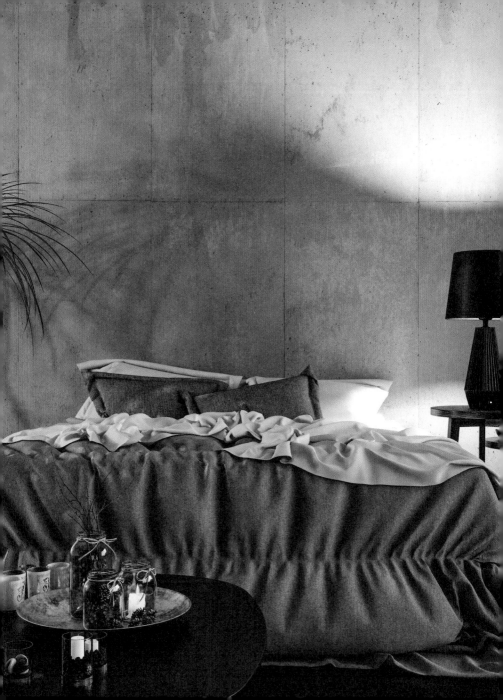

· CHAPTER TWO ·

How Sleep Works and the Role of Melatonin

Have you ever wondered *how* you actually fall asleep? Since we're not conscious when we're not awake, it's easy to feel like there's just a big blank space between going to bed and waking up in the morning.

That's far from the truth, though. As it turns out, a lot happens in our bodies—and minds—between dusk and dawn (or lights out to alarm clock).

Sleep is managed by two main systems in the body: the homeostatic system and the circadian system. The homeostatic system is a self-regulating system that helps keep your body stable and at optimal fitness for survival. A chemical called "adenosine" is the regulator in this system. The longer you're awake, the more adenosine builds up in your body. In effect, the more adenosine in your body, the sleepier you feel.

To better understand how adenosine works, consider two common forces that work for—and against—it. Physical activity boosts the level of adenosine in your body, which is why a strenuous workout makes you so tired. Caffeine, on the other hand, works by blocking adenosine, which explains how a double latte keeps you so alert.

The other system that regulates sleep-wake cycles is called the "circadian system," which works on an approximately twenty-four-hour rotation and responds to daylight and darkness in our environments. While our circadian rhythms are naturally regulated within the body, external factors—sunlight specifically—also affects them. Changing the timing of our light-dark cycles (such as working a night shift, traveling across time zones, or going through the time changes at daylight saving times), can speed up, slow down, or reset our biological clocks.

When our eyes register that the environment around us is dark, a certain group of cells in the retina known as intrinsically photosensitive retinal ganglion cells (ipRGCs)—what sleep specialist W. Chris Winter prefers to call "sleepy cells"—sends a signal to our body's "master clock." This internal clock is known as the suprachiasmatic nucleus (SCN); located in the hypothalamus, it is a small cone-shaped structure in the brain that controls many of the functions of the autonomic nervous system, including our circadian rhythms. It's the reason why you (should) feel sleepier at night and more awake during the day.

Once the SCN receives that signal, it prompts the pineal gland—a small, pea-shaped gland located just above the middle of our brain that produces and regulates certain hormones—to release melatonin, the "sleep hormone," into the bloodstream. It then circulates throughout the body, where it binds to receptors found in the pituitary gland, ovaries (in women), blood vessels, and intestinal tract. These receptors then signal to the body that it is time to sleep.

> **Melatonin** is also sometimes called the "vampire hormone" or the "Dracula hormone." Though that may sound sinister, it's not because it's evil or bad; quite the opposite, actually. Melatonin has earned that nickname simply because it *only* comes out at night.

Together, these two systems—circadian and homeostatic—work to keep our drive to sleep in check so we can be productive, alert, and energetic during the day.

Hold up. Productive? Alert? Energetic? If this doesn't sound like you in the least, don't worry. It's likely that your biological systems are working just fine. You're probably just disrupting them in some way. I'll get to the bottom of that later in this chapter.

THE STAGES OF SLEEP

Although it may not seem like it, our brains are incredibly active while we sleep. Our nightly shut-eye consists of two natural cycles of activity in the brain: rapid eye movement (REM) sleep and non-REM (NREM) sleep.

The first cycle we go through is NREM sleep, and it consists of four stages. Each of the following stages of NREM sleep lasts approximately five to fifteen minutes.

Stage 1: From wakefulness to this point in your sleep cycle, there's a 50 percent reduction in brain activity. If you're awakened during this stage while your eyes are closed, you may not feel like you've even slept a wink.

Stage 2: This is a period of light sleep with periods of muscle contractions mixed with periods of muscle relaxation. The heart rate slows, and the body temperature decreases as the body prepares to enter deep sleep.

Stages 3 and 4: These are deep-sleep stages, with stage 4 being more intense than stage 3. These stages are known as slow-wave, or delta, sleep, and they are when the body does most of the heavy lifting in terms of restoring and maintaining our general health. These stages also play a crucial role in improving our immunity and resistance to infection, which is why losing sleep can literally make us sick.

REM sleep typically begins about ninety minutes after we fall asleep. This is the period of sleep when we dream. It's characterized by certain physiological changes, including faster breathing, increased brain activity, rapid eye movement, and muscle relaxation. It's also when our brains work to store, organize, and enhance memories and learning.

During REM sleep, ideas and memories are organized into neural networks—almost like storage folders—in our brain. (This explains why pulling an all-nighter before an exam may not be the best move after all!)

How Much Sleep Do You *Really* Need?

So, how much shut-eye is *enough*?

Although this probably isn't the answer you want to hear, the most honest one is: *It depends.*

Unfortunately, humans don't come equipped with a battery icon that turns green when we're 100 percent charged. But there's a simple test you can conduct to determine whether you're getting enough sleep. Ask yourself these two simple questions from Dr. Matthew Walker:

1. After waking up in the morning, could you fall back asleep at 10 or 11 a.m.? If yes, you're likely not getting sufficient sleep.
2. Can you function optimally without caffeine before noon? If no, then you're likely sleep deprived and turning to coffee or energy drinks to self-medicate.

On the flip side, you're probably getting *enough* sleep if you feel alert all during the day, with no slump or fatigue until your regular bedtime. And if this sounds like a pipe dream, you're not alone. As the stats in chapter 1 showed, only a lucky minority of people feel this way. (Note: If you're chronically struggling with sleep, you should get a clinical sleep assessment from a sleep specialist to thoroughly address the issue.)

It's also important to note that our sleep needs change over our lifetime. According to guidelines from the National Sleep Foundation, newborns' sleep needs range from fourteen to seventeen hours (lucky them!). School-aged children should get nine to eleven hours, teenagers

DECODE YOUR DREAMS

Dreaming, which takes place during REM sleep, is how our conscious mind communicates with our unconscious mind. While interpreting dreams is not an exact science, below are possible explanations for five common scenarios you may encounter as you snooze.

Falling: Dreams about falling through the air can signify that you have fears or worries about something in your life. They can signal that you might need to change course or make a different decision about something important.

Being Chased: This might suggest a desire to escape from certain feelings that you've been trying to avoid, such as anger, desire, or fear.

Losing Teeth: A dream about missing teeth could mean that you are embarrassed about something you've done or said. It can also suggest that you are afraid of losing your ability to be assertive and self-protective.

Taking a Test: A dream about sitting down to take a test, especially one you're unprepared for, can be a sign that you're feeling stressed about an important event coming up in real life.

Infidelity: Dreaming that your significant other has cheated on you doesn't mean that this will happen or has happened. It's more likely that your brain is trying to work through another issue in your relationship, such as communication problems or an argument you and partner recently had.

Pregnancy: If you're pregnant in a dream, it's not necessarily a sign that you're with child. Instead it can suggest that you are in the midst of a creative breakthrough, or that you are strengthening a relationship with someone in your life.

need eight to ten, and adults should ideally snooze for seven to nine hours, while older adults only need seven to eight.

Finally, our sleep requirements also change according to our individual circumstances at any given time. While some of us require a full eight hours, others will be just fine on six to seven—especially if those hours are spent sleeping *well*. Finally, we may need to get more sleep during certain times of extreme stress, grief, hard work, physical training, illness, or depression.

ALL ABOUT MELATONIN

Let's dive deeper into the "vampire hormone," the sorcerer of sleep, the orchestrator of all these intriguing events, and, I assume, the reason you picked up this book in the first place: melatonin.

Melatonin was first discovered in 1958, when Yale dermatology professor Aaron B. Lerner and his colleagues isolated it in the bovine pineal gland. After finding this substance had lightened skin color in frogs, his team had been studying it in hopes that it could be useful in treating skin diseases.

However, it wasn't until 1981 that the connection between melatonin and our circadian rhythms was uncovered. That was when psychiatrist Alfred Lewy discovered that bright light at night would suppress melatonin production in humans.

In the 1990s, the hormone began to receive more attention as studies showed the effects of melatonin on sleep, as well as the potential benefits it held for other functions of the body, such as cognition and heart health. In 1994, melatonin was first sold as a dietary supplement to promote sleep.

In addition to the synthetic-supplement form, melatonin is also found in small amounts in certain foods, especially walnuts and tart cherries (either the dried version or juice). Since the amino acid tryptophan is required for the body to produce melatonin, foods high in tryptophan, such as game meat and chickpeas, are considered good sources, too. (More on this in chapter 7.)

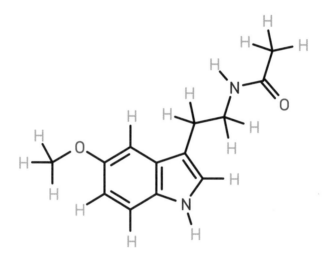

Modern Technology and Melatonin

When you read how melatonin is produced during periods of darkness, perhaps you thought to yourself, *What about all the unnatural light sources around us today? Do they interfere with our melatonin production?*

Indeed they do. In the past, our eyes would sense darkness usually a few hours after dusk, around 9 p.m. At that time, our brain would release melatonin, which would cause us to get sleepy. Melatonin levels

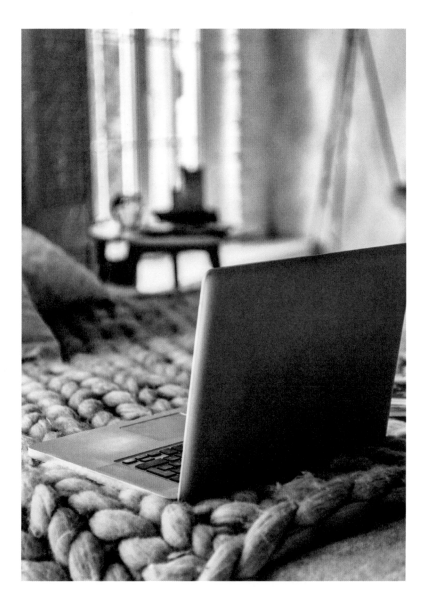

likely stayed elevated for about twelve hours, until they decreased again by around 9 a.m. During the daytime, melatonin levels are undetectable.

However, the discovery of electricity—and our always-on devices—changed all of that. (Thanks, Ben Franklin.) Artificial evening light fools our eyes into thinking that the sun has not yet set. As a result, our SCN doesn't realize it's nighttime, and won't signal the pineal gland to release melatonin.

Blue light—the type of light emitted by screens—is particularly harmful to melatonin production, suppressing its release by over 50 percent. The reason? To our brain, short-wavelength blue light appears similar to sunlight. This helps us stay awake, alert, and productive during daylight hours, but at night, it works against us. Plus, it's all around us these days—from electronics to phone screens to energy-efficient lighting—so we're exposed to more of it than ever before in human history.

In other words, your cell phone, tablet, computer, TV, and even your bedside lamp all put a hard stop on your ability to get sleepy. A study found that reading an iPad® instead of a printed book can change your sleep quantity and quality, causing people to feel less rested and sleepier the following day, and even induced a ninety-minute lag in the rise of their melatonin levels for days after—like a blue-light hangover.

Additional factors that affect melatonin production include the changing of the seasons as well as age. In the summer, when days are long, we have shorter periods of melatonin production. In the winter, when nights last longer, we produce more melatonin. Melatonin production also decreases with age, which helps explain why some people have more trouble sleeping when they get older.

Other Potential Benefits of Melatonin

In addition to melatonin's well-studied effects on sleep, preliminary research points to other possible health advantages of this hormone.

Please note that none of the following findings are conclusive, and additional research needs to be conducted. Consider the following to be *potential* beneficial effects—not absolute facts, nor reasons to take melatonin in the first place if you haven't already been doing so.

Melatonin and Cancer

One of the most exciting areas of research around melatonin is its potential anticancer effects, especially for breast and prostate cancer. Melatonin affects reproductive hormones, which helps explain why it appears to protect against cancers related to the reproductive cycle. A 2017 review of research determined that melatonin could be an "excellent candidate" for the prevention and treatment of several cancers, including breast cancer, prostate cancer, gastric cancer, and colorectal cancer.

Studies have also found that women with breast cancer tend to have lower levels of melatonin than those without the disease. Other research suggests that low levels of melatonin stimulate the growth of certain types of breast cancer cells, while adding melatonin to these cells slows their growth. Studies have shown that men with prostate cancer have lower melatonin levels than men without the disease, and one study showed that melatonin can significantly inhibit the proliferation of prostate cancer cells. Finally, some trials suggest melatonin may help reduce some side effects of chemotherapy, such as weight loss, nerve pain, and weakness, but additional trials are needed to confirm this.

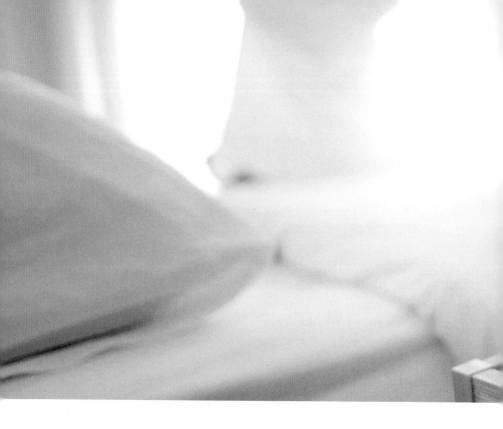

Bear in mind that these findings are *not* an endorsement of melatonin as an anticancer drug or treatment. Instead, they underline the importance of maintaining normal sleep cycles that correspond to the light and dark cycles within our environment. In fact, growing evidence points to the fact that "long-term disruptions of circadian rhythms can increase the risk of developing cancer in some individuals," as the Dana-Farber Cancer Institute reports.

In other words, you want to encourage your body to produce the right amount of melatonin for its needs. Both too much, as well as too little, of this hormone will work against you.

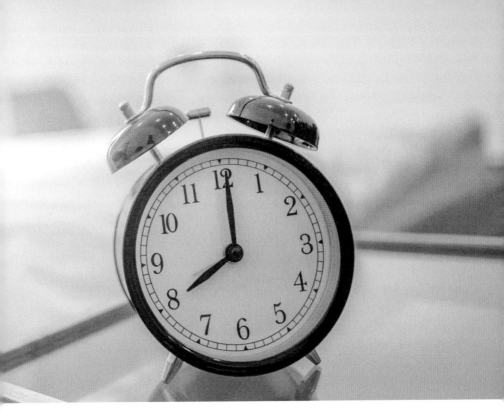

Melatonin and Cell Protection

Recent evidence has suggested that melatonin acts as an antioxidant, which means it can help fight free radicals in the body. (Free radicals are unstable molecules in cells that can damage other molecules, such as DNA, and lead to disease.) Melatonin seems to play an important role in protecting against cell damage, cognitive decline (the precursor to diseases such as Alzheimer's), and even memory loss that can arise from age and injury.

Melatonin also seems to have anti-inflammatory and antioxidant benefits for the cardiovascular system, and it may help lower high blood pressure and cholesterol. Again, this correlation needs more extensive research, but it also seems to highlight the importance our sleep-wake cycles have on our overall health, including our brain and our heart.

Melatonin's Anti-Aging Properties

Due to melatonin's antioxidant properties, it might also have potential anti-aging powers. For starters, one review of studies found that melatonin appears to have anti-aging effects on the skin, thanks to its role in protecting against UV damage to cells. Melatonin supplements have also been found to help prevent age-related bone loss, allowing people to live longer without fear of fractures or breaks to their bones. (Note that this was a study on rats, so more human research is needed.)

Melatonin and Autism Spectrum Disorders

As autism rates continue to rise, researchers are studying potential benefits of melatonin for children and adults with autism spectrum disorders (ASD). People with ASD often have trouble sleeping, and some studies have found a link between abnormal melatonin levels and the severity of ASD symptoms.

Studies have suggested that supplementing melatonin may be effective for improving sleep quality and quantity in people with ASD, and it also may help improve daytime behavior.

Melatonin and Other Medical Conditions

Although more research is needed, many studies point to additional potential uses of melatonin for issues throughout the body—from heartburn to chronic pain.

Heartburn and stomach ulcers: Several studies suggest that melatonin supplements may help treat stomach ulcers and alleviate heartburn.

Migraines: A 2019 review of studies determined that melatonin is "very likely" to be a promising treatment for migraines, although the current research is still limited.

Fibromyalgia and chronic pain: A study of people with fibromyalgia syndrome found that patients experienced a significant reduction in their fibromyalgia symptoms when they took a melatonin supplement, either alone or in conjunction with an antidepressant.

Tinnitus: Melatonin may act as a natural way to combat tinnitus, a condition that causes ringing in the ears. In a 2011 study, after taking 3 milligrams of melatonin nightly for thirty days, participants experienced a significant decrease in tinnitus symptoms as well as an improved quality of sleep.

Eye health: Thanks to melatonin's antioxidant benefits, studies suggest that it could help lower the risk of eye diseases, such as age-related macular degeneration (AMD), and help protect the retinas in patients who already have AMD.

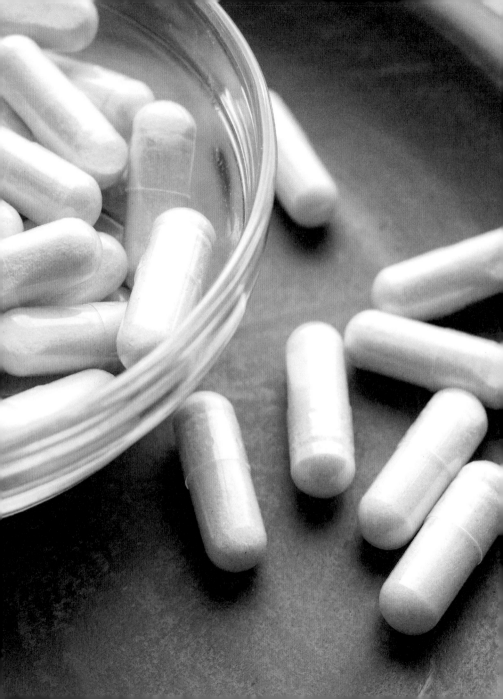

CHAPTER THREE

When—and How—to Use Melatonin Supplements

About 3.1 million American adults have tried melatonin supplements, making it the fourth most popular natural supplement on the market. Out of people who have tried a supplement for sleep, 86 percent cited melatonin as their supplement of choice. It's popular because it's available over-the-counter (in certain countries, that is—more on that shortly), non-habit-forming, and since our bodies already produce it naturally, well, it seems safe.

Before I get into what melatonin supplements *can* do for your sleep, let's get one thing out of the way: Melatonin supplements are *not* sedatives. As discussed in the previous chapter, melatonin is a natural hormone released by your brain that signals it's time to go to sleep. Translation: It doesn't help you *stay* asleep, but plenty of evidence points to the power of melatonin to help you fall asleep—fast.

WHY USE MELATONIN SUPPLEMENTS?

A meta-analysis of nineteen studies on sleep disorders found that melatonin supplements helped reduce the time it took to fall asleep by an average of seven minutes. In many of these studies, people also reported a significantly better quality of sleep.

Melatonin supplements can be especially helpful for people experiencing disruptions in their circadian rhythms, such as those working night shifts or traveling across time zones. Since melatonin helps signal to your body that it's dark outside and it's time to go to sleep, it helps you reset your internal body clock to get you back on a regular sleep schedule.

Melatonin supplements have been shown to help reduce jet lag by syncing your internal clock with the time change. One analysis of ten studies deemed melatonin supplements to be "remarkably effective" at reducing the effects of jet lag, and found "occasional short-term use" to be safe. The researchers also found that both lower doses (0.5 milligram) and higher doses (5 milligrams) were equally effective at reducing jet lag.

It also comes in handy for people with a condition known as delayed sleep phase syndrome. Adults and teens with this sleep disorder have trouble falling asleep before 2 a.m. and have trouble waking up in the morning. In a 2007 review of the literature, researchers suggested that a combination of melatonin supplements, a behavioral approach to delay sleep and wake times until the desired sleep time is achieved, and reduced evening light may even out sleep cycles in people with this syndrome.

Melatonin is also proven to help older people, who may be producing lower levels of natural melatonin, get better sleep. A 2012 study looked at the effects of 2 milligrams of prolonged-release melatonin supplements in the treatment of insomnia in patients fifty-five years or older. The trial found the supplement helped improve sleep quality and length, morning alertness, and participants' health-related quality of life when compared to a placebo pill. The study author also found no dependence, tolerance, or withdrawal symptoms.

Melatonin supplementation has also been indicated as a sleep aid that can help offset the side effects of menopause. In one study of perimenopausal and menopausal women, most women taking the supplement reported better sleep as well as general improvement of mood, and found that it significantly mitigated depression associated with menopause.

Melatonin supplements can play a useful **short-term** role in helping a variety of people get better sleep. In addition to people struggling with jet lag or taking on shift work, melatonin can also help almost anyone gradually reset their bedtime in order to wake up earlier.

CHOOSING A SUPPLEMENT

Melatonin supplements can typically be found in tablet, chewable, or gel-capsule form. In the US, they're available over-the-counter at pharmacies, supermarkets, and health-food stores, but in other countries, they may require a prescription. Originally, melatonin supplements were derived from the pineal glands of animals, but today, most melatonin supplements are synthesized in labs.

Sourcing Melatonin

In the US, melatonin supplements are the only hormone that can be purchased without a prescription. Since it's considered a dietary supplement, it isn't regulated by the same safety or efficacy standards that the Food and Drug Administration (FDA) sets for over-the-counter (OTC) medications and prescription drugs. It's also available over-the-counter in Canada, but in the European Union, New Zealand, Australia, and some other countries, you need a prescription from your doctor to buy melatonin. There are, however, some lower-dosage versions that you may be able to find on the shelves or buy online, usually labeled "circadian tablets."

To ensure you're getting a quality product, look for "pharmaceutical grade" printed on the packaging. Also, in the US, check that the product has been approved by a supplement-verifying organization such as ConsumerLab.com, NSF International, U.S. Pharmacopeia, or UL. This can provide some assurance that a product isn't contaminated, and it contains what's listed on its label.

Unfortunately, there's still a chance that the supplement label isn't fully accurate. An investigation at the University of Guelph, located in

Ontario, found that in more than 71 percent of melatonin supplements, the amount of melatonin was more than 10 percent different from what the product label indicated. Some products contained as much as 478 percent more melatonin than advertised. Do some research online with a supplement-verifying organization, such as the ones listed previously, to ensure you're choosing a high-quality, reputable brand, or check with your doctor or pharmacist if you're not sure about which brand to get.

HOW TO TAKE MELATONIN SUPPLEMENTS

The best time to take a melatonin supplement is thirty minutes to one hour before bedtime. If you're traveling and taking it for jet lag, take it ninety minutes before you go to sleep in your new destination. Also, try to get at least twenty minutes of sunlight in the morning—whether you simply open your curtains or head outside for a walk—to help reset your internal clock.

Start with the lowest possible dose, and don't overdo it. (See the list below to find the starting point for your particular need.) Experts say that doses should not exceed 10 milligrams per twenty-four hours, and they warn against increasing your dose without consulting your doctor. If melatonin helps you sleep better one night and then doesn't work as well the next, it doesn't mean you should up your dose and start taking more.

Here are the doses recommended for certain sleep conditions, based on scientific studies:

- For regulation of sleep-wake cycles: 0.3–5 milligrams
- For insomnia: 2–3 milligrams
- For jet lag: 0.5–8 milligrams, starting upon day of arrival at destination
- For delayed sleep phase syndrome: 3–5 milligrams

The most important thing to keep in mind about melatonin supplements is that they're intended for short-term, transient sleep issues. The National Institutes of Health have deemed melatonin to safe to use for three months, but research hasn't examined whether it continues to be safe if used for longer than that.

If you feel the need to take melatonin supplements for longer than three months—or to take it every night—it's time to take a step back and consider seeing a specialist to get to the root of your sleeplessness.

Possible Side Effects and Interactions

A 2005 meta-analysis determined that melatonin supplements are generally safe for healthy adults to use for three months or less. They come without the addictive nature and dangerous side effects of prescription-strength sleep aids, such as next-day drowsiness, heartburn, headaches, stomach pain, and sleepwalking (or even sleep-driving!).

However, melatonin supplements can have some mild side effects, including headache, dizziness, and stomach irritation or cramping. Less common side effects include short-term depression, irritability, or confusion.

Some people also report having "crazy" dreams while taking melatonin. Experts, however, are not certain that melatonin specifically causes this phenomenon, since there may be an increase in REM sleep with melatonin, and vivid dreams occur during REM sleep.

Pregnant and breastfeeding women should not take melatonin supplements. People with the following health conditions should exercise caution and be sure to check with their doctors before taking melatonin supplements:

- Bleeding disorders
- Depression
- Diabetes
- High blood pressure
- Seizure disorders
- Organ transplant

If you use sedative medications, such as Klonopin®, Ativan®, or Ambien®, do not use melatonin supplements. They may also interact with medications, as well as:

- Anticoagulants and antiplatelet drugs
- Anticonvulsants
- Contraceptive drugs
- Diabetes medications
- Medications that suppress the immune system (immunosuppressants)

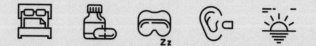

6 THINGS TO KNOW BEFORE TAKING MELATONIN SUPPLEMENTS

1. Talk to your doctor first.

Always consult your physician before you begin taking a supplement or make any changes to your existing medication and supplement routine. As such, please consider the information in this book not as medical advice, but as information to potentially start a conversation with your doctor. Pregnant and breastfeeding women should not use melatonin. People with bleeding disorders, depression, diabetes, high blood pressure, or seizure disorders, as well as transplant recipients should exercise caution and absolutely must check with their doctors before taking melatonin.

2. It's best to use in the short-term—not the long run.

Similar to a bandage or a brace, melatonin supplements should be considered a temporary—rather than long-term—solution. Plus, it is highly unlikely that anyone has a melatonin deficiency, so it's not a medically necessary supplement.

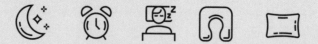

3. Obtain your supplement from a quality, safe source.

Go for the synthetic form of melatonin supplements, which are less likely to be contaminated than those sourced from an animal. Also, look for "pharmaceutical grade" printed on the packaging as well as a seal by a supplement-verifying organization.

4. Take the right amount at the right time.

Start with the lowest possible dose at least thirty minutes prior to bedtime.

5. Check for interactions with medications.

Ask your doctor about any potential interactions between melatonin and any medications you're taking.

6. Be aware of possible side effects.

Melatonin supplements can have some mild side effects, including headache, dizziness, and stomach irritation or cramping. Less common side effects include short-term depression, irritability, or confusion.

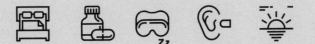

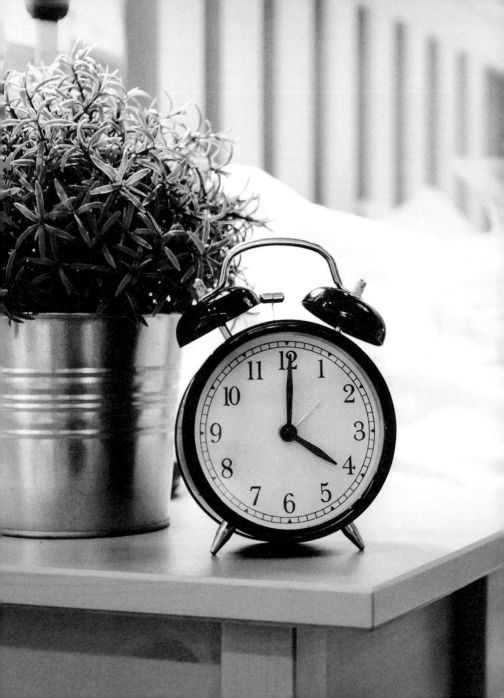

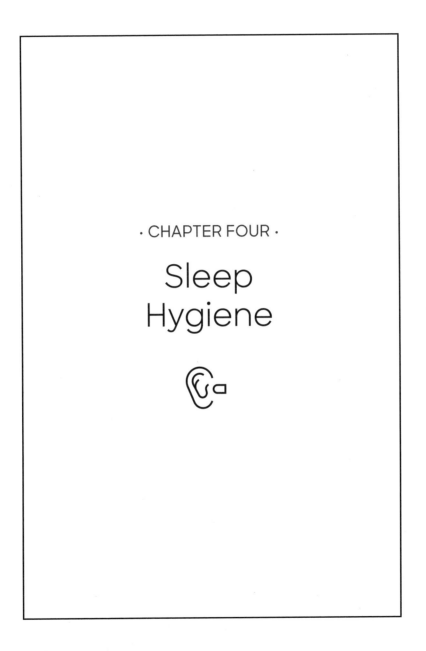

· CHAPTER FOUR ·

Sleep Hygiene

Now that we have a better idea of the power of sleep, how it happens, and the mechanisms of melatonin, let's dive deeper into the best sleep tips and practices. I know what you might be thinking, *Wait a second. I bought this book to find out how melatonin can help me sleep—not to be told I have to change my entire nighttime routine!*

Here's the thing. While melatonin is certainly an important—and natural—piece of the puzzle for a good night's sleep, it's far from a be-all and end-all solution. A supplement that you have to take every night, natural or not, should always be a short-term fix, rather than a long-term solution. Plus, since its long-term effects haven't been fully researched yet, experts recommend only using it for three months at most, as discussed in chapter 3.

In order to sleep better in the long run—while improving your health, well-being, work, *and* relationships—you're going to have to make a few changes in the way you approach sleep and your nighttime habits. What the research shows (and what I've personally found to be true) is that sleep hygiene, as well as certain science-backed routines, can make a big difference in helping you catch better zzz's.

Luckily, making these changes doesn't have to be hard. I've experimented with many—if not all—of the following tips, and it's been so much easier than I expected to adjust my sleep environment and integrate new habits into my nightly routine. And the payoff is so worth it. Without a doubt, implementing these changes has changed my sleep—and my life—for good.

WHAT IS SLEEP HYGIENE?

Let's begin with the basics. Although it sounds like a euphemism for a private bathroom behavior, *sleep hygiene* actually refers to "the act of controlling your sleep behaviors and environments in an effort to optimize your sleep," as sleep specialist W. Chris Winter describes it.

Essentially, sleep hygiene encompasses all the things that you *can* control to set yourself up for a successful night's sleep. And it turns out there's quite a lot within your control.

In this chapter, I'll categorize the best sleep-hygiene habits according to the five senses: sight, sound, touch, smell, and taste. Looking at your bedroom through the lens of your five senses can help you evaluate your environment and create your very own sensory-friendly, sleep-inducing haven.

Sight

The most important environmental change you can make for better sleep is to make your bedroom dark, and I mean really, *really* dark.

The signals that your eyes take in directly affect your biological clock (remember the SCN?), which tells you what time to go to sleep and what time to wake up. Your body naturally produces melatonin in the evenings to help you fall asleep, but this will *only* occur if your eyes can't see light. In other words, the light in your bedroom, or lack thereof, can mean the difference between lying awake and staring at the ceiling at 2 a.m. or being blissfully unaware in dreamland. In fact, *any* source of light—whether it's your phone screen, a sliver of light peeking beneath the door, or the LED numbers on your clock—can prevent your brain from producing melatonin.

As I talked about in chapter 3, the most villainous kind of light is blue light, so here are some ideas on how you can combat the effects of blue light and all light sources in general.

Power down an hour before bed. In an ideal world, you'd leave your smartphone, tablet, laptop, and other electronic devices out of the bedroom—completely. In a realistic world, you should stop staring at them at least sixty minutes before bedtime. Surprisingly, this also includes e-readers. According to a 2014 study, people who used e-readers before sleep took an average of ten minutes longer to fall asleep and experienced less REM sleep than individuals who read a printed book with indirect light.

Can't quit your electronics at night? Hey, I get it. You can still take some measures to decrease the amount of blue light you're getting, such as installing an app on your smartphone or computer that reduces the amount of blue light the screen emits at night. You might also want to consider buying blue-light-blocking glasses, which are hitting the mainstream market in droves these days.

Charging my phone in the kitchen or the bathroom, rather than on my bedside table, has been a game-changer for my own sleep habits. If you need an alarm in the bedroom, invest in an inexpensive, old-fashioned alarm clock—just make sure it doesn't tick. But if the clock has LED lights, cover the display with a pillowcase, or consider wearing a sleep mask to block it out. Even those glowing numbers can be a hindrance to the total darkness your brain craves at night.

Install blackout shades. Or at least choose drapes in a dark fabric to block out ambient light from outside. If your curtains or drapes are dark but don't stay closed very well, there's a simple solution. Grab a large chip clip (yes, the kind from the kitchen!) and use it to secure the sides of each drape together to prevent any light from peeking through the openings between them.

Wear a sleep mask. A comfortable sleep mask can work wonders if you have sources of light you just can't prevent from coming through—such as a partner who gets up before you or who just can't quit watching late-night TV. Look for a thick one with space for your nose and a strap that you can secure tightly around your head, so it doesn't fall off in the middle of the night.

Lower your wattage. Consider swapping your regular lightbulbs for natural-light, 45-watt bulbs. About an hour before bedtime, dim all light sources to produce less than 200 watts total. If your partner likes to read at night, ask him or her to use a small book light.

Choose the right hues. Of course, our eyes take in more than just light and darkness. The way our bedrooms *look* can also make a key difference between poor sleep and wonderful, peaceful shut-eye, so decorate your bedroom with the right colors. Bright hues like red or orange, for example, can evoke panic and drama, not exactly what you want in a relaxing environment.

Instead, opt for soothing color schemes, neutral shades like beige or cream (white can be too stark and clinical), or pastels like pale greens, blues, and yellows. For wall decor, choose pleasing images that help you relax, rather than stimulate you—think flowers, trees, or peaceful landscapes.

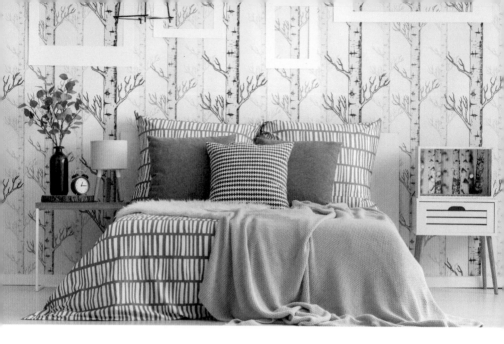

Tidy up! A messy room can have an effect on your subconscious, promoting a sense of worry that impedes your ability to sleep. So, tune in to your inner Marie Kondo and get to work: clean out your closet, pick up and put away all clothing, and be sure to leave any work-related supplies (computer, printer, files) out of the bedroom. The last thing you need while you're drifting off is a reminder of the presentation that Bob needs on his desk at 9 a.m. next Monday.

Sound

After sight, sound is the second most important sense in terms of sleep. Whether it's a snoring partner, a noisy heating system, or ambient noises from outside, here's how to take a stand against noise in the bedroom.

Play some noise. If your nights are anything but silent, a white-noise machine might become your new best friend—it's certainly become mine. I've found I cannot sleep without white noise, whether it's from an app on my phone, a machine, or a fan.

While it sounds counterintuitive to add noise to your environment, these machines emit a soft, static-like sound that's scientifically shown to help drown out unwanted sounds and promote better sleep. You can purchase a white-noise machine online, but there are cheaper alternatives. For instance, you can buy a small fan or leave your ceiling fan on at night if it makes enough of a whirring noise. Or if you have a clock radio in your room, set it between two stations for a soothing static. You can also download white noise apps on your phone, but as I discussed, it's better to keep electronics out of the bedroom.

Tune in and zone out. Prefer to have something in your ears that you can actually listen to? This is an instance where it might be OK to keep your smartphone in your room. Some apps offer premade playlists full of soothing tracks intended to help you wind down at night, and you can even find libraries of relaxing "sleep stories"—basically bedtime stories for adults. If you share your bed with someone, be considerate and use earphones to listen, so you don't mess with their sleep!

Plug it in. Finally, if you prefer absolute silence (and don't mind sleeping with something stuck in your ears), earplugs are a good option. Look for a pair that have *NLR* (noise-level rated) on the label, which means they are effective at reducing ambient noise.

Touch

Imagine the coziest, dreamiest place you've ever slept. A place where falling asleep felt simple, where you felt so relaxed you could drift off almost instantly, where the bedding was so delicious it felt as if you were lying on a cloud.

Now, let's make your bed that very place. Yes, you might have to spend a bit of money to make this happen, but you don't have to spend a fortune.

Buy the best bedding. For the ultimate sleeping sanctuary, purchase the most comfortable sheets, pillows, and mattress cover you can afford. Ask your friends, read reviews online, and find the best sleep accessories for you. If you come across one you love at a hotel, check the brand and then buy it for yourself.

Here's some good news: You don't have to buy some crazy-high thread count sheets. While a 400 thread count sheet is finer and softer than a 200 thread count sheet, anything above 400 is probably not going to be that much better or worth the money.

Get a cozy pillow to rest your head on. Try out several different types in a store (if possible) to decide for yourself which softness you prefer. While there's no right or wrong choice, there are certain suggestions based on your sleeping style. For example, a firmer pillow works well for side sleepers, flatter pillows help support head-and-neck alignment for on-the-back sleepers, while stomach sleepers might prefer a very soft pillow.

Finally, you don't have to rush out and buy a new, expensive mattress. An affordable pillow-top mattress cover can make a big difference. However, if you've used the same mattress for more than seven years, it's probably time for a new one.

Lower the thermostat. Before bedtime, don't forget to lower the thermostat. Experts say that the ideal sleeping temperature is between 65 and 72 degrees Fahrenheit (18 and 22 degrees Celsius). If you tend to get hot at night, you can look into a cooling mattress or point a small fan at your side of the bed. If you get cold at night, consider getting a heavier duvet, flannel sheets, or even a heated blanket to help you stay warm. I've found that a heavy comforter adds a sense of security and helps me feel super calm and cozy as I fall asleep, too!

Dress down. When it comes to pajamas, less is more. Opt for loose-fitting, light sleepwear. You can always put on extra layers, but it's more disruptive to have to rip off that sweatshirt in the middle of the night.

Warm up before bed. To further relax and ease tight muscles, try taking a hot bath or shower right before bed. The subsequent drop in body temperature after the warm water evaporates from your skin has been proven to help induce feelings of sleepiness.

Beware of bedmates. One final thing that many of us "touch" at night: another body! Some of us sleep with our pets or even our children in bed with us. While there are different schools of thought on this subject, the general rule of thumb is that if your kids or pets don't disturb your sleep (or your partner's), there's usually no harm in letting them share the sheets.

If, however, Fido's snoring constantly wakes you up or your child is interrupting your sleep (or your intimacy!), then it might be time to reconsider. Talk to your family doctor for more advice.

Smell

Your olfactory system (sense of smell) is powerful, and odors can greatly impact how fast you fall asleep—and how well you sleep overall.

Select some sleep-inducing scents. Science has shown that certain smells not only lift your spirits but also possibly reduce anxiety, agitation, and even pain—all good for inducing sleep. The most soothing scents include lavender, rose, vanilla, and chamomile, while more energizing smells, such as peppermint or lemon, should be avoided right before bed.

Reap the benefits of aromatherapy by using essential oils (either infused into the air via a diffuser or rubbed on the skin), putting on scented body lotions, spritzing a linen spray on your bedding, or bringing in some fresh flowers or live plants.

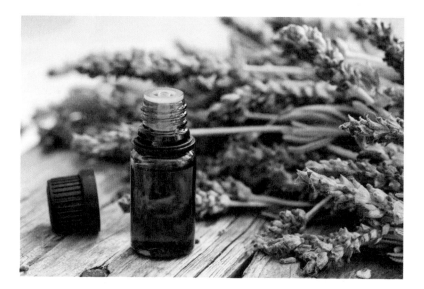

Change your sheets. Wash your bedding at least once a week using hot water and a hypoallergenic detergent to keep your bed smelling nice and fresh. Body odor, as well as dirt and bacteria, can build up on sheets faster than you think.

Light a candle. If the glowing flicker and soothing scent wafting from a candle puts you at ease, go for it. Just be sure to blow it out before falling asleep, and follow the additional safety tips below.

CANDLE SAFETY TIPS

- When blowing out a candle, make sure that the wick ember is completely out and no longer glowing.
- Keep candles away from household items that could catch fire, such as drapes, bedding, or books.
- Cut the wick down to about ¼ inch (6 mm) every time before burning. Longer wicks can lead to uneven burning and dripping, which can increase the risk of a fire.
- Stop using a candle when it gets close to the bottom of the container or holder.
- Avoid burning candles too closely to each other; keep them at least 3 inches (7.5 cm) apart.
- Watch out for air currents from drafts, vents, or ceiling fans—these could lead to uneven burning or flare-ups.

Taste

Last but not least, the foods you eat and beverages you drink before you get in bed can play a crucial part in your sleep-hygiene habits. What's more, the timing of when you have certain foods and drinks is also significant when it comes to getting good sleep.

Unsurprisingly, there's a fairly lengthy list of what you should avoid. However, just as if you were trying to eat healthier, try not to focus on what you're "supposed to" eat or drink. Instead, I'd suggest that you focus on what you *can* eat and drink—and there's plenty to choose from, as you'll see in the final chapter of this book.

Cut back on caffeine. It should come as no surprise that caffeine has a detrimental effect on our sleep. It can both reduce slow-wave sleep—the most restorative kind—and also decrease overall sleep time.

People differ greatly in their physiological responses to caffeine. While it's typically excreted from the bloodstream within a few hours of consumption, the exact amount of time depends on age, weight, gender, hormones, and metabolism. For older people, it may take longer (up to twenty hours!) to metabolize caffeine.

Because of this, there's not a cut-and-dried time to stop consuming caffeine, but experts typically recommend cutting off caffeine consumption by 2 p.m.—if not earlier. And don't have too much, no matter how early in the day. The National Sleep Foundation considers six or more 8-ounce cups (240 ml) of coffee to be an "excessive" intake.

Don't worry; I'm not trying to take away your coffee completely. Coffee has plenty of benefits, such as increasing alertness, concentration, and even boosting your mood. You don't have to cut it out altogether. Just be sure to keep in mind the timing and potential downsides of your daily java, along with the perks.

Avoid alcohol. As with most things we consume to "help us sleep," alcohol produces sedation, not necessarily good, solid sleep. While a glass of wine or two may make us fall asleep faster, this doesn't necessarily translate into better sleep, or improved performance the following day. Plus, as the alcohol metabolizes during the second half of the night, it can cause wake-ups (often to pee), dry mouth, headaches, and more disturbances that worsen the quality of your sleep.

Ideally, you'd cut out alcohol entirely in favor of more solid sleep. But if you're going to imbibe, experts suggest you stop drinking at least two hours before bed and stick to only two drinks. The reason being that one serving of alcohol takes about one hour to metabolize, so if you have two drinks, they'll "wear off" by that time.

Dine on the early side. Avoid eating large meals within three hours of bedtime. If you're trying to digest food while you're trying to settle into a slumber, your body will find it difficult to handle both of these processes simultaneously—and neither process will go smoothly.

Snack smartly. If your stomach starts rumbling right before bed, it's OK to have a snack—just make sure it helps, not hinders, your sleep. Keep it around 200 calories, and try to eat it at least an hour before your actual bedtime. (Lots of tasty examples can be found in chapter 7!)

The perfect bedtime snack combines complex carbs and protein. Including some calcium in the form of dairy in your bedtime snack is also smart, because calcium helps the brain convert the amino acid tryptophan (found in many proteins) into melatonin. Combined with carbs and protein, calcium also helps your brain produce serotonin, known as the calming hormone.

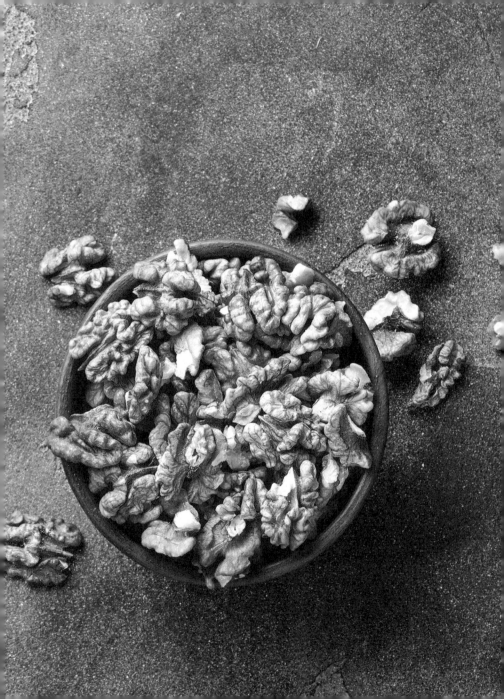

There are a few foods that contain melatonin itself—most notably, walnuts and tart cherries. While the amount found in those foods isn't enough to make a huge difference in your sleep, they can enhance your body's own melatonin production process. Other sleep-inducing ingredients that are ideal for your bedtime snacks include:

- Foods high in tryptophan, such as lean proteins, game meat, and chickpeas
- Foods high in magnesium, such as almonds, dairy, and leafy greens like kale
- Foods high on the glycemic index, such as bananas, dried fruit, and cereal
- Dairy foods high in calcium, such as yogurt, milk, and cheese
- Teas with calming ingredients, such as chamomile, lavender, passionflower, and valerian

Know your no-goes. Unfortunately, that tasty Thai takeout isn't the best choice before bed. In addition to caffeine and alcohol, try to avoid spicy or super garlicky foods at night, which can cause sleep-disrupting digestive issues. Also avoid consuming foods that are particularly high in fat (such as fried foods, burgers, ice cream, or heavy pastas) right before bed.

The reason? Foods high in fat take the longest to digest—up to six hours! Foods high in protein tend to move through your digestive tract more quickly, and carbohydrates pass through the fastest, which is why carb-centric snacks are ideal for nighttime nibbles.

Finally, don't drink too much of anything once you finish dinner. A cup of calming tea is great, but even that should be in moderation. Your body takes ninety minutes to process liquids, so ingesting lots of liquids close to bedtime can cause middle-of-the-night bathroom trips.

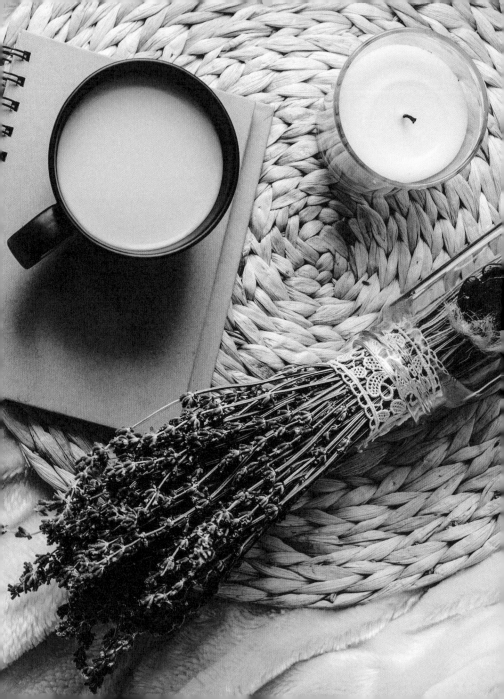

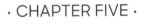

· CHAPTER FIVE ·

Bedtime
Rituals

Once you have the basics of sleep hygiene dialed in, the next step is to create a consistent bedtime routine. Our bodies like to follow familiar patterns at night, which signal to our biological clocks that it's time to wind down and get ready for sleep.

You probably already have a semblance of a nightly routine that you stick to, such as cleaning up the kitchen, washing your face, and brushing your teeth. Perhaps you've even added melatonin supplements to your list of nightly tasks.

Now, it's time to add something a little extra. Consider these rituals as more than just extra "to-dos," but part of your self-care routine. *Self-care* has become a big buzzword in the wellness world, and while you may have some vague idea that it involves bubble baths and face masks, self-care is about much more than that. At its core, self-care means shifting your mind-set away from what you have to do—for your family, for work, for other people—and focusing on what *you* need in the moment. Although that may sound selfish on the surface, it's quite the opposite.

Having go-to self-care rituals, such as the ones that follow, will enable you to be your most productive, energetic, and all-around happiest self, which in turn helps you be more present and helpful to others. Self-care has also been shown to help boost your mood, increase productivity, curb sugar cravings, and—you guessed it—promote sleep.

Consider these the missing piece of the puzzle, in addition to melatonin supplements you might be taking. Just remember, there's no one-size-fits-all approach to relaxation. Just as someone loves cycling classes when another person dreads them, not everyone's idea of "relaxing" is going to look the same. Treat this list as an all-you-can-eat buffet of sleep-inducing rituals, and pick and choose what appeals to you.

1. Tap into your motivation. It may sound a little out there, but the first step to getting a good night's sleep is to dig into your *why*—the deep-down reason you want to sleep better in the first place. Adapting to new habits and routines can be hard, but when you tap into your self-motivation, change will feel a lot easier. In other words, whatever is important in your life should serve as motivation for you to commit to changing your sleep for the better.

To find your why, ask yourself the following questions: *What motivates me to get up each morning? What is missing from my life that more sleep could help me cultivate? Why do I want to have more energy during the day—to do a hard workout, to tackle a business project, to play with my children? Why is that important to me? What is the worst-case scenario if I don't change my sleep habits? What is the best-case scenario if I improve my sleep habits?*

You'll want to figure out your why as you begin to work toward better sleep and then you can turn to your answers or ask yourself these questions again whenever you need a refresher as to *why* you're working to improve your sleep habits. When you adopt a purposeful, motivated approach like this, changing your habits will become a lot more doable— and your results will be a lot more likely to last.

2. Sip some tea. Not only is the act of brewing a fresh cup of tea relaxing in itself, but certain types of tea come with calming properties proven to help you get ready for sleep. Studies have shown that chamomile tea has antianxiety benefits, while valerian root tea has sedative properties that can decrease the time it takes you to fall asleep. Other teas with proven benefits for sleep include passionflower, lavender, peppermint, rose, and lemon balm.

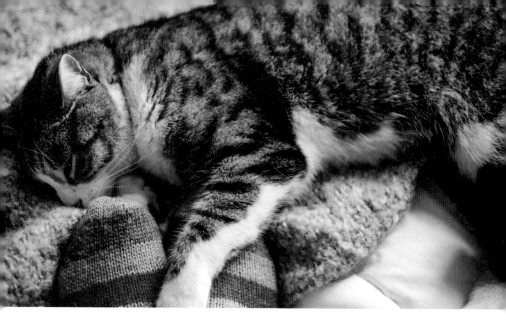

3. Cuddle up. Being close to your spouse, partner, child, or even a pet can boost levels of oxytocin, the "love hormone." Oxytocin has been shown to reduce stress levels, improve mood, and enhance sleep. Just a simple kiss good night and a wish for sweet dreams can work wonders to create a cozy mood before bed.

4. Take your vitamins. Swallowing vitamins is an excellent bedtime ritual that serves as a signal to wind down, benefits your well-being, and even may improve your sleep. Invest in a good multivitamin that contains these vitamins and minerals, all of which have been shown to aid sleep:

- B vitamins: These vitamins play a crucial role in helping your body process and use the energy it receives from food.
- Calcium: Not only does this nutrient benefit your bones but it is also an important factor in the conversion of the amino acid tryptophan into melatonin.

- Magnesium: Magnesium is an important nutrient for many processes in the body, such as regulating muscle function and stabilizing blood sugar. Research suggests that it helps to enhance deep sleep and can also help people having trouble sleep get better shut-eye.
- Zinc: A naturally occurring mineral in the body, zinc has been shown to play a critical role in shortening the time it takes to fall asleep and increase sleep quality.

5. Stretch it out. Prepare your body for sleep with a few stretches or yoga poses that can help soothe anxiety: cat/cow, downward-facing dog, forward fold, and legs-up-the-wall are particularly relaxing poses.

On the following pages, Ava Johanna, a Los Angeles–based yoga and meditation instructor, shares a beginner-friendly ten-minute yoga routine you can do before bed. Just grab a mat and do these moves right beside your bed so you can doze off when you finish!

6. Try progressive relaxation. If doing a whole yoga routine sounds like a bit much, don't sweat it. In this exercise, all you have to do is lie still. It also works wonders to help soothe an anxious mind and tense body.

- Lie on your back and close your eyes.
- Starting with your forehead, focus on tensing and then relaxing every single part of your body. Tense and soften your forehead, eyes, face, jaw, neck, and so on, continuing to move each body part, one at a time, until you reach your toes.
- When done, surrender to gravity, feeling your bed fully support your weight. Stay in this relaxed state for a few minutes, focusing on your breath and releasing all other concerns.

A 10-MINUTE BEDTIME
YOGA ROUTINE

1. Child's Pose (Minutes 1–3)

This pose stretches the shoulders and chest while opening the hips and lower body.

How to: Spread your knees wide but keep your big toes touching. Sit your hips back onto your heels and crawl your palms forward until your forehead rests on your mat. Start to connect to your breath by noticing the length of your inhale and exhale. Use your inhale to crawl the palms an inch farther and use your exhale to sink the hips even deeper toward the heels. Optionally, rock your forehead side to side to massage the space between your brows.

2. Cat/Cow Pose (Minutes 3–4)

This transitional pose opens the spine, shoulders, and chest.

How to: Come down to all fours on your hands and feet—this is the table-top position. Stack your shoulders above your wrists and hips above your knees. Keep your gaze down and slightly forward so the spine and back of the neck remain long. On an inhale, roll the shoulders down your back and press your chest forward. On an exhale, tuck your chin toward your chest and lift the back of your heart high. Continue alternating between these movements for one minute, elongating your inhale and exhale to create more space in the spine.

3. Downward-Facing Dog (Minutes 4–5)

This gentle inversion elongates the spine and helps realign the vertebrae.

How to: From tabletop position, tuck your toes and lift your hips up and back to come into an inverted V shape. Spread your fingertips wide, with your middle fingers pointing forward. Keep your feet hip width apart or wider and find a gentle bend in the knees. On your inhale, lift your hips and lengthen your spine. On your exhale, bring your heels closer to the mat.

4. Forward Fold (Minutes 5–6)

This pose opens the lower back, hamstrings, and calves while releasing tension along the spine.

How to: From downward-facing dog, step your right foot, then left foot, up to your palms. Bring your big toes in to touch and find a slight bend in your knees. Keep your palms on the mat, or clasp the backs of your calves to bring your torso closer to your thighs. Maintain the bend in your knees, draw your belly button in toward your spine, and then relax your head, neck, and shoulders.

5. Standing Folded Twist (Minutes 6–7)

This pose opens the hamstrings, IT (iliotibial) band, and lower back.

How to: Start standing with your feet hip width apart. Fold over your legs, keeping a generous bend in both knees. Center your left palm between your feet and reach your right palm toward the sky, opening your chest toward the right. If accessible, start to straighten your right leg for more of a stretch in the lower back and IT band of the right leg. After a few breaths, switch sides.

6. Supine Twist (Minutes 7–9)

This pose decompresses and realigns the spine while opening the chest.

How to: Lie on your back and inhale as you pull your right knee into your chest. Your left leg will stay long with toes flexed up toward the sky. As you exhale, shift your right leg across the body so the knee gently drops toward the left side of your body. Extend your palms in opposite directions while keeping your shoulder blades firmly pressed into the mat. After a few breaths, switch sides.

7. Legs-up-the-Wall Pose (Minutes 9–10)

This pose increases circulation by facilitating lactic acid drainage in the lower body.

How to: Bring your hips against the wall or your headboard in bed. Walk your feet up the wall and bring the sit bones an inch closer to the wall until your body is in an L shape with your feet extended toward the sky, taking slow, deep breaths for one minute.

8. Savasana . . . or Sleep!

This final pose facilitates deep relaxation, preparing your body for sleep.

How to: Allow the entire back of your body to rest heavy on the mat beneath you. Place your palms face up toward the sky and widen your feet to hip-width distance. Your toes will naturally drop out to the side. You can also practice this pose in bed, so you can stay in savasana for as long as you need until you are ready to sleep.

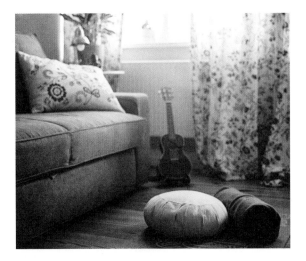

7. Breathe deeply. Your breath is intricately connected to your nervous system, which means that taking long, slow breaths can literally slow down a busy mind. Studies have shown it can improve mood and reduce stress and anxiety—all keys to getting a good night's sleep.

To harness the relaxing power of your breath, begin by doing the progressive relaxation exercise described in step 6. Then add on this breathing exercise:

- Inhale slowly through your nose, feeling your lungs fill with air and your belly extend outward. Breathe in slowly, over a count of eight to ten seconds.
- Hold your breath at the top for a second or two.
- Quietly and easily relax and exhale, squeezing all of the air out of your lungs.
- Wait a couple seconds, and then repeat the cycle.
- Ideally, this will take you right to dreamland after a few cycles.

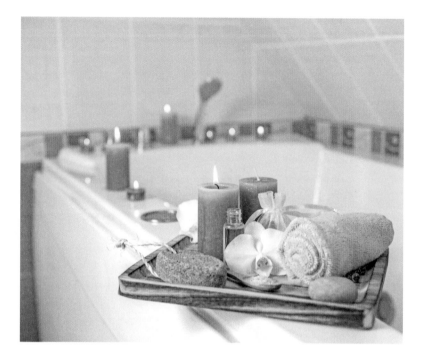

8. Take a hot shower or bath. As I mentioned in the last chapter, warming up and then lowering your body temperature before bed has been proven to help you feel sleepy. Go for a warm soak in the tub or take a hot shower. If you're lucky enough to have access to one, hit the hot tub!

9. Experiment with essential oils. As I mentioned in the last chapter, your sense of smell plays a powerful role in helping you sleep—but just make sure you're using the right kinds of oils *and* in the right way. Choose scents that have calming properties such as lavender, bergamot, sandalwood, rose, and clary sage.

According to experts, the best way to reap the benefits of essential oils is by breathing in the scents. You can use a diffuser or place oils in a personal inhaler, or on a cotton ball, or simply rub them on your skin. (Be sure to check the label to ensure the formula is intended for that use, and skip essential oils if you have pets at home—certain essential oils, especially tea tree oil, can be poisonous to our four-legged friends.)

10. Play some mind games. No, not the kind your ex played with you. Instead, I'm talking about guided imagery and little mental games that can help you detach from the day, soften your focus, and even "trick" your mind into falling asleep fast. Here are a few examples to try out from Dr. Michael Breus, also known as The Sleep Doctor:

- Imagine you are a sponge lying in a pool of warm water. Pretend that the pores of your body are like the pores of a sponge. As you breathe in, you are drawing in this warm, relaxing water through every pore of your body. Feel the warmth penetrate your skin. As you breathe out, the water is soaking into every pore of your body. Focus on the feelings of heaviness and warmth. Continue breathing in and out, imagining the water filling in all the nooks and crannies.
- Picture being in your favorite, most relaxing place in the world. Maybe it's a sunny beach where you're swinging in a hammock as the warm breeze caresses your skin and hair. Maybe it's on top of a mountain, looking out over a vast landscape. See if you can conjure up exactly how your surroundings look, feel, sound, and smell.
- Imagine you're standing in front of a chalkboard. On the board, write down all those pesky thoughts that are interrupting your

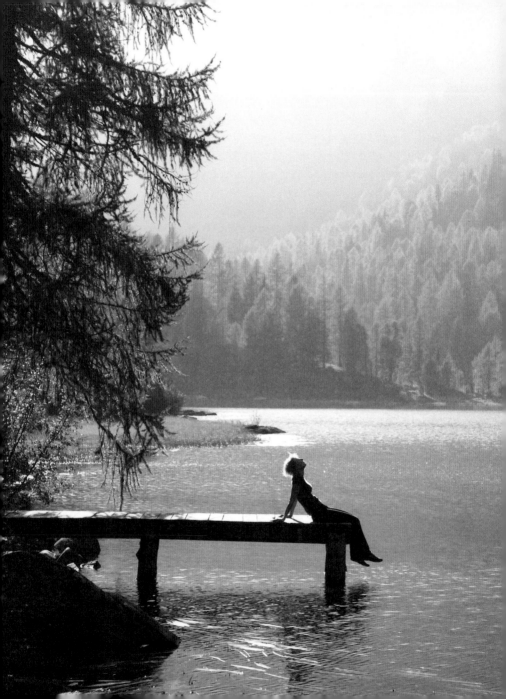

sleep. Now, erase them all. Admire the clean, blank board, continuing to stare at it while keeping your mind blank as well.

- Work your way through the alphabet from A to Z and come up with four- or five-letter words beginning with each letter.
- Imagine you're describing your hometown or neighborhood in the greatest possible detail to a stranger.

11. Bring some "hygge" into your life. I already covered tips to make your bed the most comfortable sleep sanctuary ever (see page 46). To take it a step further, add in a bedtime ritual inspired by the Nordic concept of *hygge* (pronounced hoo-gah), which loosely translates to a "cozy way of life."

At its roots, this Nordic tradition is about getting back to basics, prioritizing what's important, and simplifying your life. To bring some hygge into your life, brew and sip a cup of warm tea before bed, or read by candlelight (keep it safe by being sure to blow out the candle before you go to sleep). Of course, do all of this while wearing your coziest set of pajamas. Bonus points for fuzzy socks.

12. Listen to soothing music.
Lullabies aren't only for little kids. Consider making a calming playlist full of chill tunes that help you wind down. You can also turn to music services for playlists with sleep-friendly songs.

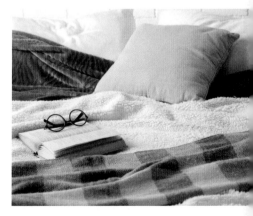

13. Choose calming content. Right before bed is not the time to read a heart-pumping adventure or watch a violent horror movie. Stick with more soothing stories for your bedtime reading (think biographies, self-development tomes, or chick-lit books). If you must watch TV, stick to shows that are on the more boring side, like period dramas rather than crime shows.

Also, consider limiting your intake of news at night, and focus on reading or watching content that evokes feelings of calm and well-being—not anger or frustration, like the news tends to do these days!

14. Meditate. Meditation has become one of the most-talked-about wellness trends in recent years, and it's been linked to improved sleep and reduced insomnia in several studies.

But what is meditation, really? To the uninitiated, it may just seem like sitting in silence, not thinking about or doing anything. That's sort of right, as meditation is essentially a state of stillness where no effort is necessary.

Through that stillness, however, meditating helps you cultivate a deeper awareness of your body and mind. It helps you notice how your body feels and become aware of the passing thoughts and feelings in your mind. Eventually, it helps to change how you view—and how you react to—the many thoughts, feelings, and emotions that pass through your mind.

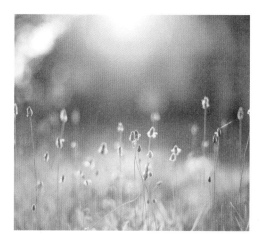

STEPS FOR MEDITATING

To try out a basic meditation, follow these guidelines. You can also download one of the many free or paid meditation apps that will walk you through basic, beginner-friendly meditations.

1. No need to sit cross-legged on the floor. Simply find a place that's comfortable to sit in for a few minutes, whether it's a couch, a chair, or a cushion. Keep your back straight yet relaxed, chin slightly tucked, and rest your hands lightly on your lap or knees.
2. Close your eyes and relax all your muscles, beginning with your feet and progressing to your face.
3. Stay relaxed. Choose a calming focus, such your breath going in and out. You can also choose a word or phrase (such as *relax* or *peace*) that you can repeat aloud or silently as you inhale or exhale.
4. Let go and relax. Don't judge yourself or worry about how you're doing. When you notice your mind has wandered, simply take a deep breath and gently return your attention to your chosen focus.
5. Continue for ten to twenty minutes. When finished, sit quietly with your eyes closed for a few minutes, then open your eyes for a few minutes before standing up.

15. Pick a mantra or affirmation. Repeating a mantra can be the perfect complement to your nighttime meditation practice. You can choose a phrase, such as "I am relaxed," or go with a Sanskrit mantra that is known to calm and balance the mind for sleep, such as *sa ta na ma*. These sounds mean "birth, life, death, and rebirth" and are said to help wake us to our divine nature. You can also try using a sleep-focused affirmation, such as "I welcome deep, satisfying sleep," or "I will wake up refreshed and energized."

16. Write down your worries. Journaling can work wonders to calm a worried mind. Buy a small notebook and pen to keep beside your bed. Every night when you get in bed, write down whatever is stressing you out—from personal problems to to-do lists to work issues. Try to include at least one potential solution for each one, even if it's "deal with it tomorrow."

Then, close the journal, signifying that you're done worrying about it for the night. You can also jot down any troublesome thoughts (or strokes of genius!) that pop into your mind in the middle of the night in the journal too.

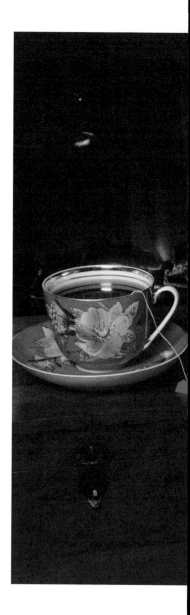

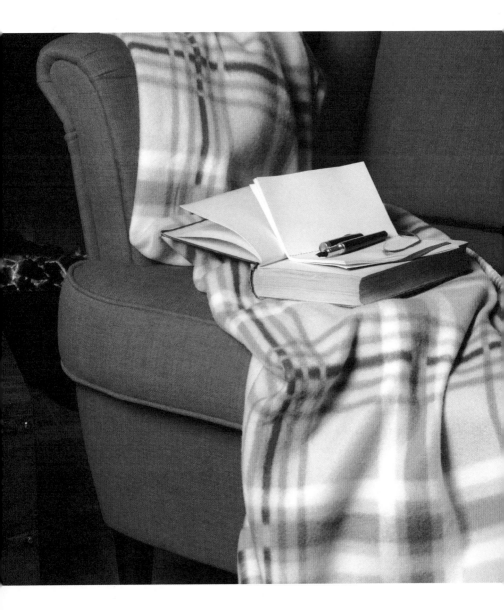

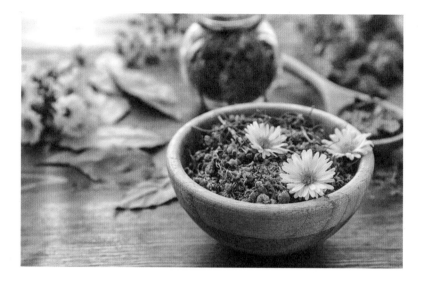

17. Eat (and drink) wisely. Refer to page 53 for a full list of no-no's to avoid before bed. But, if you're hungry and you need a snack before you sleep, certain foods and combinations of foods can help you get some solid shut-eye. In chapter 7, I'll share twenty delicious sleep-inducing recipes that are easy to make during your nightly routine.

18. Stick to a schedule. Having a nighttime routine is not the only factor that should stay consistent. Your bedtime and wake-up time should also be pretty much set in stone—yes, even on weekends! If you simply must sleep in, don't sleep for more than an hour past your weekday wake-up time.

The reason? Regularity is essential for setting and stabilizing your internal sleep-wake biological clock. Plus, maintaining a regular sleep schedule will make you feel significantly more alert, and within a few weeks it can actually reduce the total sleep time required for full-day alertness.

What's more, if you sleep in on the weekends, you might find yourself dealing with Sunday-night insomnia. This means you may not be able to fall asleep until after midnight, and then before you know it, your alarm goes off, starting your workweek off on a bad note that can lead to a vicious cycle. In fact, it's like you've given yourself jet lag without even leaving home. If you do end up staying up later than usual on any given night, aim to get up the next morning at the usual time to prevent this cycle from setting in.

19. Set an intention to wake up energized. This has been a huge realization for me recently. You can actually influence the way you feel in the morning by setting an intention before you go to sleep. For example, I've experimented with telling myself, "I will wake up with energy and excitement to take on my day." And guess what? I do.

Intention setting in this way can "trick" your mind into feeling more awake in the morning, thanks to the powerful mind-body connection— the idea that the thoughts and beliefs in our minds can positively (or negatively!) influence our physical health. In other words, mind over matter can really work!

20. Stop trying so hard. After all that advice, sometimes the best thing to do is just to *relax*. Trying to force the issue is one of the worst things you can do, because it can lead to anxiety around bedtime, which can in turn make your sleep even worse.

If you find falling asleep to be impossible, the best thing to do is get up, go to a quiet area of your house, read a book, do some light housework, crochet, or paint. When you feel ready to fall back asleep, head back to the bedroom, and chances are good sleep will be much more likely to head your way.

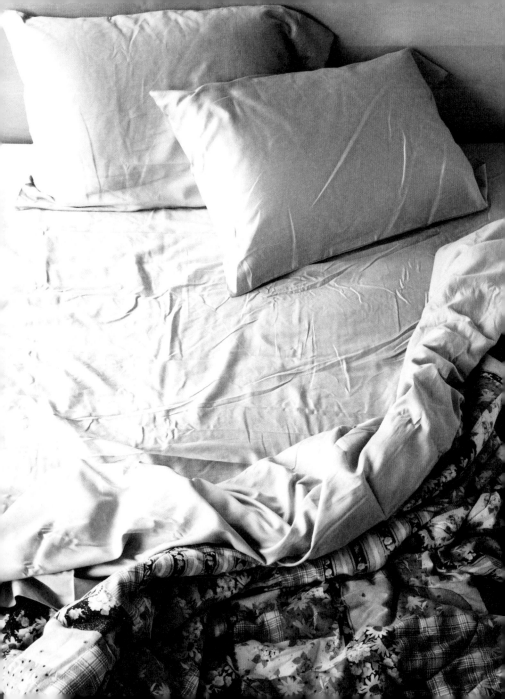

CHAPTER SIX

The Five-Week Plan to Upgrade Your Sleep—and Your Health

Now, it's time to put everything you learned on the previous pages together.

Following this five-week program will help you create an ideal sleep environment in your bedroom and establish a personal list of helpful, sleep-inducing bedtime rituals that work for you. You can do this program whether or not you're taking melatonin, but if you are using melatonin supplements for a short period of time, this is a wonderful way to create long-term sleep habits that will stay with you for life.

Each week, you'll set three sleep-related goals: finding your ideal bedtime, implementing changes to improve your sleep hygiene, and trying out a new bedtime ritual. Basically, this plan offers a practical way to sift through all the information you've learned so far in this book and put it into action. I've also included a chart on pages 80–81 where you can track and keep a record of all your work.

By the end, you will have discovered the habits, tips, and tricks that enable you to fall asleep fast, sleep more soundly, and wake up feeling more refreshed than ever before. Just remember to be patient. Your sleep hygiene and habits took years to get to where they are now; it'll take more than one night to fix them.

Note: The following program is five weeks long, but if a five-week plan sounds a little unwieldy—or you just want to sleep better ASAP—you can shorten it to three weeks by integrating the sound and touch sleep-hygiene changes into the second week, and combining smell and taste in the third week. Just pick one bedtime ritual to try each week for a total of three.

Week 1

Goal 1: Focus on finding your ideal bedtime. Set what time you want to get up—and count backward eight hours! If you find it takes you a while to fall asleep, count back nine hours.

Here's where technology is your friend: many smartphones nowadays have a "bedtime" alarm clock where you can set an alert to remind you to start getting ready for bed.

Goal 2: Starting with the sense of *sight,* follow the tips on pages 41–44 to improve your sleep-hygiene habits and environment. (I suggest starting with sight, since that's the most important sense for sleep.)

Goal 3: Pick one of the rituals in the last chapter to start integrating into your bedtime routine. It doesn't matter which one; just pick one that appeals to you. If it doesn't work out after trying it out at least two times, that's fine—move on to the next one that you like! The whole goal is to figure out which bedtime rituals work best for *you,* not to impose any new routines you'll dread doing every night.

Week 2

Goal 1: Keep your bedtime and wake-up time consistent. You might still be trying to figure out exactly how much sleep you need, and it's OK if you need to keep experimenting. The catch? Keep them the same on the weekends! If you simply must sleep in, don't do so for more than an hour past your weekday wake-up.

Goal 2: Focus on the sense of *sound*, and follow the tips on pages 44–45 to ensure a quiet and peaceful sleep environment.

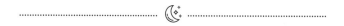

Goal 3: Pick a second ritual to add into your bedtime routine, while keeping the one you chose in week one. Again, play around if the first one you choose doesn't seem to jibe with your nightly routine. This should be a cumulative process of adding in a new ritual each week.

Week 3

Goal 1: Continue keeping your bedtime and wake-up time consistent. When you feel like you've hit your sleep sweet spot, try experimenting by cutting fifteen minutes off your sleep time and see if that makes you feel drowsy the next day—if not, then you know you've found your ideal personal sleep requirement.

Goal 2: Tackle the sense of *touch*, and make some of the recommended adjustments on pages 46–47 to your sleep environment.

Goal 3: You guessed it—pick a third ritual to add to your bedtime routine. Remember, changing your mind is A-OK!

Week 4

Goal 1: Still keeping your bedtime consistent? Fantastic! If not, recommit to staying on track with your timing.

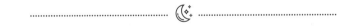

Goal 2: Time to focus on your sense of *smell* by following the recommendations on pages 48–49.

Goal 3: Choose a fourth ritual for your nightly routine.

Week 5

Goal 1: You should basically be a sleeping machine by now.

Goal 2: Last but not least, it's time to focus on sleep hygiene surrounding food and drink with the tips on pages 50–53. To treat your taste buds, I recommend trying some of the sleep-promoting bedtime snacks in the next chapter!

Goal 3: Pick the fifth and final ritual to add to your bedtime routine. You should now have an enjoyable, and doable, five-step routine that you look forward to doing every night!

SLEEP TRACKER

Copy this chart to track how your new habits affect your sleep over these five weeks. If you're finding patterns—either positive or negative—after certain rituals or changes to your environment, adjust accordingly. Each week you'll be figuring out what works and what doesn't!

Week: _____

Bedtime: _____

Sleep-Hygiene Habits: _____

_____

_____

Date	Lights-Out Time	Time It Took to Fall Asleep (Approx.)	Wake-Up Time

New Bedtime Ritual: _____

_____

_____

Additional notes or reflections:

_____

_____

_____

_____

_____

Quality of Sleep (on a scale of 1–10)	Energy and Mood in the Morning (on a scale of 1–10)	Energy and Mood in the Evening (on a scale of 1–10)	Melatonin Supplement Usage (Y/N)

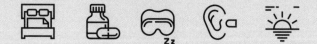

HOW TO BECOME A
MORNING PERSON

Not an early bird? You're not alone. Studies suggest that only around 18 percent of people are truly "morning types," while 27 percent are "evening types." Morning types tend to go to sleep earlier and feel their best in the mornings, while evening types stay up later and perform better in the afternoon. Your chronotype—aka whether you're a morning or evening person—is determined by your genes.

The good news: No matter your chronotype, you can make some tweaks to your routine and environment to become more of a morning person, even if it's not in your genetic makeup. Here are a few simple changes you can make tonight.

Get enough sleep.

The first step to becoming a morning person begins the night before. One hour before your ideal bedtime, turn off your screens to avoid melatonin-suppressing blue light, try out some of the bedtime rituals in chapter 5, and start preparing for bed.

Look forward to your morning.

Give yourself a reason to hop out of bed. Maybe that reason is a freshly brewed cup of coffee or taking a walk somewhere truly beautiful. Or

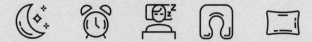

maybe you want to use some of that extra time in the morning to start a side hustle or that novel you've always wanted to write. No need to wait until Friday to get excited; once you find your reason to wake up, I guarantee that getting out of bed will feel a lot easier.

Prepare for the day ahead.
Before you go to bed, check your calendar so you know what's coming up the next day, jot down a to-do list if you're stressed, and if you're planning to exercise in the morning, lay out your gym clothes the night before so they're easy to slip on.

See the light.
Open all the blinds as soon as you wake up if the sun is out, or turn on the lights if it's still dark. When your eyes see bright light first thing in the morning, it helps shut down melatonin production and reset your internal clock, helping it get used to getting up earlier.

Move your body.
Exercising first thing in the morning can help you get in gear for the rest of the day. If getting up and getting to the gym sounds like torture, try doing a ten-minute yoga routine or a bodyweight workout in your living room. A quick search online will turn up plenty of options.

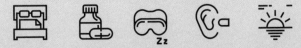

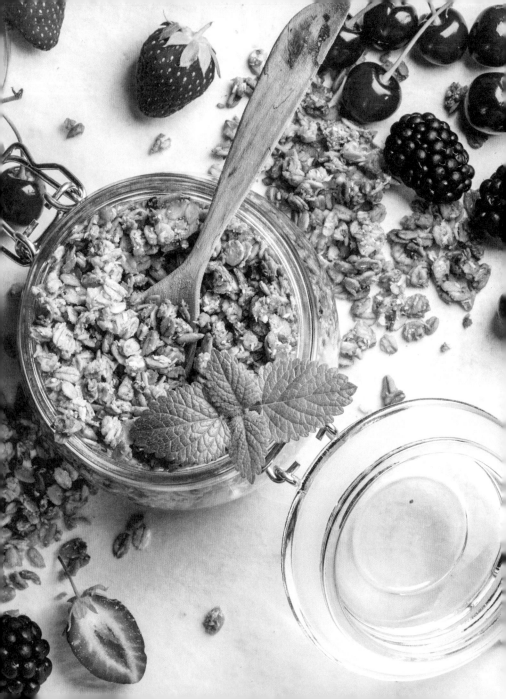

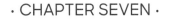

· CHAPTER SEVEN ·

Bedtime Snacks
for Better Sleep

The relationship between food and sleep can be a double-edged sword. As I covered on page 53, certain foods can disrupt your sleep, most notably spicy dishes or foods that are high in fat. On the other hand, many delicious—and healthy—ingredients have been scientifically shown to support a good night's rest. This chapter has twenty tasty recipes that are all simple to make and include foods that can help boost your melatonin levels and promote better sleep.

Melatonin, as you know by now, is a natural hormone secreted by the pineal gland. A few foods also naturally contain melatonin and can modestly boost our body's production of melatonin, and you'll find many of those foods in the recipes in this chapter. But keep in mind that melatonin levels are much more impacted by light, as described in chapter 4.

While there's no one single food you should eat to boost your melatonin production, researchers recommend eating a healthy diet in general, one that's rich in vegetables, fruits, and whole grains. The variety of minerals and nutrients you get from eating nutritious foods like those helps contribute to the overall synthesis of melatonin.

There is one ingredient in particular that can help improve our melatonin levels: tryptophan, an essential dietary amino acid that's a precursor to melatonin production. Tryptophan can be found in most protein-rich foods, especially chicken, turkey, eggs, cheese, fish, seeds, nuts, and legumes. See the list on the next page for more foods that can help support sleep.

COMMON SLEEP-INDUCING FOODS

Bananas
Grapes*
Strawberries*
Kiwi
Dried fruits
Avocado
Leafy greens*
Tomatoes*
Sweet potatoes
Almonds**

Chickpeas*
Cherries and
   cherry juice*
Chicken**
Turkey**
Eggs*
Greek yogurt**
Cacao**
Sunflower seeds***
Pistachio nuts***

Walnuts*
Nut butters**
Almond milk**
Dairy**
Herbal teas (decaf)
Whole grains**

---

*contains melatonin
**contains tryptophan
***contains melatonin
   and tryptophan

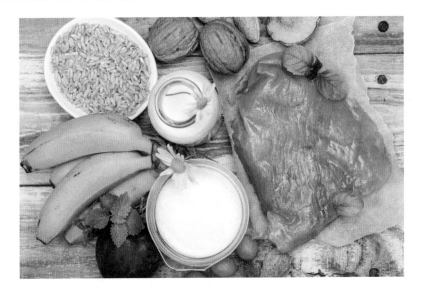

ROMESCO RICOTTA TOAST

Sleep-inducing foods: tomato, walnut, bell pepper, whole wheat, dairy

YIELD: 2 SERVINGS

Sweet and savory romesco—a sauce made from tomatoes, roasted red peppers, and toasted walnuts—is delicious on pasta but also makes a great late-night snack when simply spread on toast. Here, it's paired with creamy ricotta on a slice of toasted whole-wheat bread, which is just rich enough to satisfy those pre-bedtime munchies without feeling like you've eaten another meal. Save any leftover sauce (or double the recipe) for dinner tomorrow night.

INGREDIENTS

Romesco sauce:

1 tablespoon tomato paste

¼ cup (85 g) roasted red peppers from a jar

1 small garlic clove

1 tablespoon lemon juice

¼ cup (30 g) toasted walnuts

1 tablespoon extra-virgin olive oil

Freshly ground black pepper

Kosher salt

2 slices whole-wheat bread

¼–⅓ cup (62–82 g) ricotta

Lemon zest, optional

DIRECTIONS

- Combine the tomato paste, peppers, garlic, lemon juice, and 3 tablespoons of the walnuts in a food processor or blender until smooth. With the motor running, slowly pour in the olive oil. Season with salt and pepper to taste. Crush the remaining walnuts and set aside.

- Toast the bread in a toaster or in the oven. Let cool slightly, then spread each slice with half the ricotta, making a slight well in the center of each. Fill the wells with prepared romesco sauce. Top with the remaining crushed walnuts and lemon zest if using; season with more salt and pepper.

- Store leftover romesco sauce in a sealed container in the fridge for up to one week.

RAINBOW FRUIT SALAD

Sleep-inducing foods: orange, kiwi, peach, pineapple, pomegranate

YIELD: 2–4 SERVINGS

Most fruit salads are hastily tossed together in a bowl using past-their-prime berries and mushy stone fruits. Not the case here! This bright and zippy plate of orange, kiwi, peach, and pineapple is drizzled with a lime-ginger dressing, which brightens up the fruit flavors. This dish is finished with salt, pepper, and a glug of olive oil, which might not be your first instinct when it comes to fruit, but these seasonings actually make the fruit taste more like itself, adding a depth of flavor most fruit salads sorely lack.

INGREDIENTS

1 orange

1 lime, zested and juiced

1 teaspoon grated fresh ginger

Kosher salt

1 kiwi, peeled and cut into thin slices

1 peach, cut into wedges

¼ fresh pineapple, peeled and cut into rough 1–inch (2 cm) chunks

2 tablespoons pomegranate seeds

Black pepper

Extra-virgin olive oil

DIRECTIONS

• Halve the orange crosswise and juice one half into a small bowl. Peel and slice the remaining orange into wedges and place in a shallow bowl. Whisk the lime juice and ginger into the orange juice. Season with a pinch of salt.

• Combine the kiwi, peach, and pineapple with the orange slices. Pour the dressing over the fruit. Top with the lime zest, pomegranate seeds, black pepper, and a drizzle of olive oil.

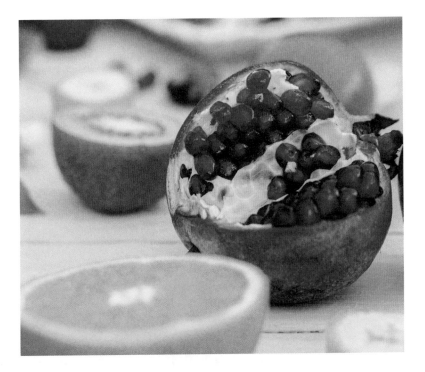

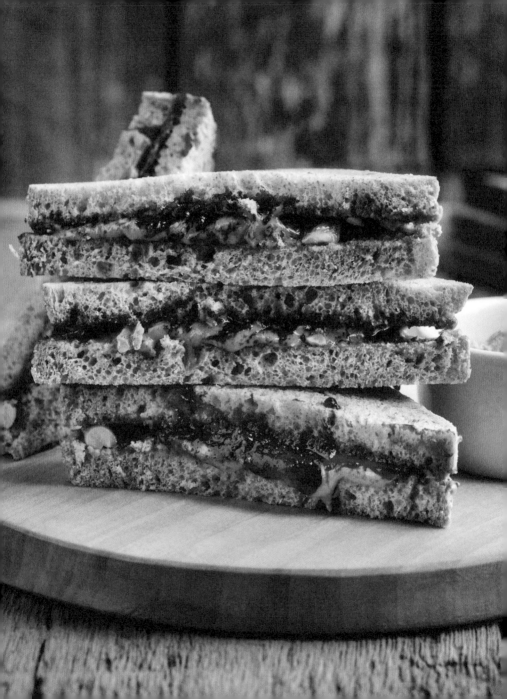

SLEEPY PB&J (PISTACHIO BUTTER AND GRAPE-CHERRY JAM TOAST)

Sleep-inducing foods: grape, tart cherry, pistachio, whole wheat

YIELD: 1 SERVING, PLUS EXTRA JAM AND NUT BUTTER

Pistachio butter can be pretty expensive at the store, but luckily it's a snap to make yourself. Just plan on standing next to the food processor for a while; it can take a good ten to twenty minutes to get a really smooth pistachio paste. And nothing goes with DIY nut butter like homemade jam—this one is a sweet-and-sour mix of red grapes and tart cherries. Smear both spreads over a slice of whole-wheat toast and you've done it: a perfect PB&J for those in their pj's. A note on tart cherries: fresh ones are hard to find year-round; a good alternative is to buy them canned—stored in water, not syrup.

INGREDIENTS

½ pound (227 g) seedless red grapes

1 cup (155 g) tart cherries, pitted and halved

½ cup (64 g) granulated sugar

2 tablespoons lemon juice

½ cup (62 g) toasted unsalted pistachios, shelled

¼ teaspoon cinnamon

2 slices whole-wheat bread

Flaky sea salt, optional

DIRECTIONS

• Roughly chop the grapes. Combine the grapes, cherries, sugar, and lemon juice in a medium saucepan. Over medium heat, stir until sugar is dissolved. Bring the heat up to medium high and cook until the mixture comes to a boil. Boil for five minutes, skimming off any foam that rises to the top. Reduce heat to medium low and simmer, stirring occasionally and breaking up the fruit with the back of a spoon, until the mixture has thickened, about twenty minutes. Let cool.

• While the jam is simmering, combine the pistachios and cinnamon in a food processor and pulse until the mixture gets crumbly. Scrape down the sides of the bowl and grind until the mixture forms a thick, smooth paste (this can take up to twenty minutes, depending on the strength of your food processor), scraping down the sides again as need be. You can also make this in a high-power blender, which should take about ten minutes.

• Toast bread in a toaster or in the oven. Let cool slightly, then spread one slice with 2 tablespoons of the pistachio butter. Spoon 2 tablespoons grape-cherry jam over the nut butter. Top with flaky sea salt if using. Place the remaining slice on the spreads to assemble the sandwich.

• Store remaining jam and nut butter in the fridge; use the jam within two weeks and nut butter within three months. As the jam tends to firm up a bit when chilled, bring it to room temperature or reheat it on the stove to loosen it after refrigeration.

AVOCADO-CACAO MOUSSE

Sleep-inducing foods: cacao, almond milk, avocado

YIELD: 2 SERVINGS

Yes, you read that correctly: avocado and chocolate. You probably won't find this one on a dessert menu at your average restaurant, but when mixed with melted chocolate and maple syrup, buttery avocado blends into a mousse worthy of any fancy French bistro. To top it off, add a handful of toasted almonds for a bit of crunch.

INGREDIENTS

2 ounces (57 g) bittersweet chocolate, chopped

2 tablespoons room-temperature almond milk

1 avocado, halved and pitted

1–2 tablespoons maple syrup

1 tablespoon cacao powder or cocoa powder

½ teaspoon vanilla extract

Kosher salt

Flaky sea salt, optional

Almonds, chopped and toasted, optional

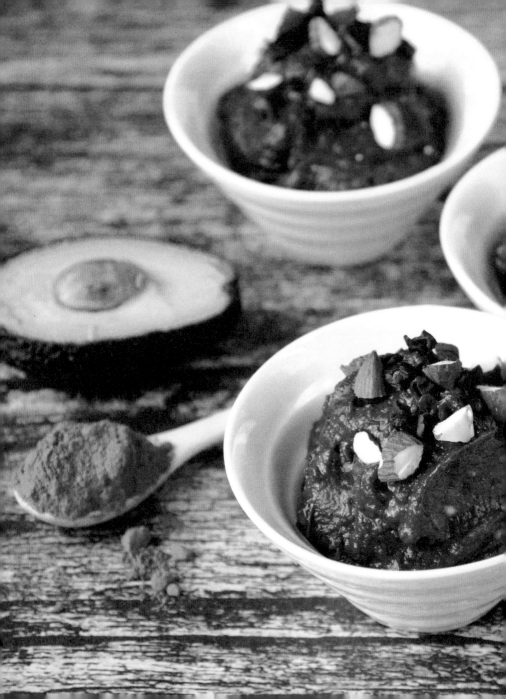

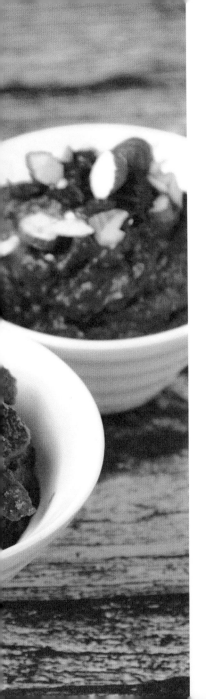

DIRECTIONS

• Melt the chocolate in a heat-proof bowl in the microwave or over a double boiler. Let cool slightly and whisk in the almond milk.

• Combine the cooled chocolate mixture, avocado, 1 tablespoon maple syrup, cacao powder, vanilla extract, and kosher salt in a food processor or high-power blender. Blend until smooth. Taste and add the second tablespoon of maple syrup if desired.

• Divide the mousse into two cups. Serve immediately, or refrigerate for at least two hours (or up to overnight) for a thicker consistency. Before serving, top with a pinch of flaky sea salt and toasted chopped almonds if using.

SALTED HONEY NUT CHEWY GRANOLA BARS

Sleep-inducing foods: almond, walnut, pistachio, almond butter, oat, flaxseed, tart cherry

YIELD: 16 SERVINGS

Consider this recipe the final reason to stop buying granola bars at the store. Honey and almond butter act as the glue for a mixture of almonds, walnuts, pistachios, and chewy dried tart cherries. Plus, you've got oats and flaxseed in there for some added protein, fiber, and omega-3 fatty acids. The result? A sticky, crunchy snack that tastes better (and is better for you) than any bar you can get in the cereal aisle.

INGREDIENTS

¼ cup (38 g) raw almonds

¼ cup (30 g) raw walnuts

¼ cup (31 g) raw pistachios

½ cup (125 g) unsweetened almond butter

¼ cup (85 g) honey

½ teaspoon kosher salt

1 cup (90 g) rolled oats

2 teaspoons ground flaxseed

¼ cup (40 g) dried tart cherries

DIRECTIONS

• Line an 8 × 8–inch (20 × 20 cm) baking pan with parchment paper, allowing for a 2-inch (5-cm) overhang and set aside. Preheat the oven to 325°F (160°C). Spread the almonds, walnuts, and pistachios on a sheet pan and toast for ten to fifteen minutes, tossing occasionally, until they are golden and fragrant. Set aside to cool.

• In a medium saucepan, combine the almond butter, honey, and salt over medium heat until the mixture becomes runny, about three minutes. Whisk the melted mixture into a smooth, runny nut butter. Remove from heat.

• Roughly chop the cooled nuts and add to the almond butter mixture along with the oats, flaxseed, and tart cherries.

• Press the mixture into the prepared baking pan. Cover with another piece of parchment paper. Refrigerate for at least one hour to set. Remove from the pan by lifting the edges of the parchment paper. Cut into sixteen pieces.

• Store bars in a sealed container in the refrigerator for up to one week, or in the freezer for three months.

Note: Feel free to customize the recipe by adding in your favorite mix-ins, such as raisins, dried blueberries, sunflower seeds, or chopped pistachios.

Salted Honey Nut
Chewy Granola Bars

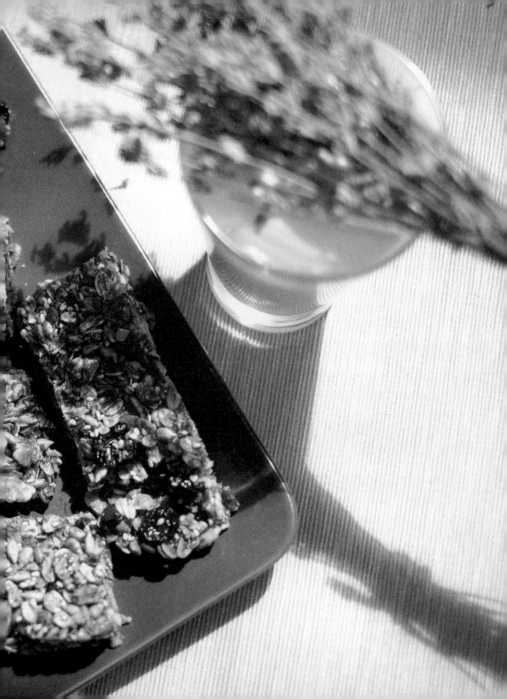

CHERRY-AND-RICOTTA PARFAITS

Sleep-inducing foods: tart cherry, orange, dairy

YIELD: 2 SERVINGS

If you're not macerating fruit, you're missing out. When mixed with sugar (or another sweetener like maple syrup or honey) and orange juice, tart cherries soften and sweeten into a juicy mixture you'll want to put on everything—and why shouldn't you? Here, the cherries are layered with a blend of ricotta and Greek yogurt, for a tart and creamy dessert that lies somewhere between a yogurt parfait and a sundae.

INGREDIENTS

½ cup (78 g) tart cherries, halved and pitted

1 tablespoon granulated sugar, maple syrup, or honey

½ orange, zested and juiced

¾ cup (168 g) ricotta

¼ cup (56 g) low-fat Greek yogurt

Extra-virgin olive oil, for drizzling

Flaky sea salt

DIRECTIONS

• Combine the cherries, sugar, orange zest, and orange juice in a small bowl. Cover and chill for at least one hour or up to overnight. Drain liquid.

• In a small bowl, whisk together the ricotta and yogurt.

- Spoon 2 tablespoons cherry mixture into the bottom of two 4-ounce (120 ml) glasses. Spoon ¼ cup (56 g) yogurt mixture over the cherries. Repeat with another layer of cherries and yogurt. Top with a drizzle of olive oil and a pinch of flaky sea salt.

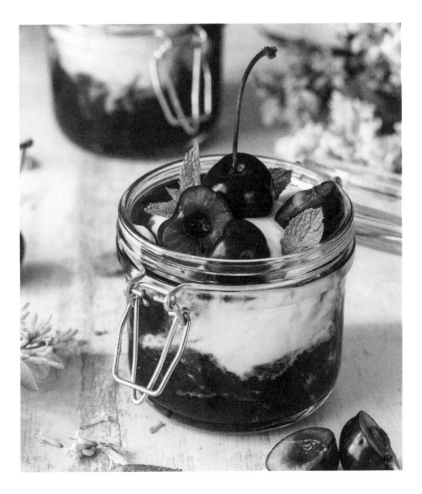

DATE-AND-NUT BITES

Sleep-inducing foods: oat, walnut, cacao, flaxseed, dried fruit, almond butter

YIELD: 18 SERVINGS

Sticky-sweet dates and toasted nuts are a match made in heaven. And while you could snack on them straight from the container at the end of the night, these bites are a slightly more composed alternative. Feel free to swap in toasted almonds or pistachios for the walnuts, or try peanut or sunflower-seed butter instead of the almond butter. The only non-negotiable? The crunchy, chocolaty cacao nibs on top.

INGREDIENTS

3 tablespoons rolled oats

⅓ cup toasted (40 g) walnuts

3 tablespoons cacao powder or cocoa powder

½ cup (40 g) shredded unsweetened coconut

3 tablespoons ground flaxseed

½ teaspoon kosher salt

½ teaspoon cinnamon

10 pitted dates, soaked in hot water for fifteen minutes

¼ cup (63 g) unsweetened almond butter

1 tablespoon almond or oat milk

1 teaspoon cacao nibs

DIRECTIONS

• Line an 8½ × 4½–inch (22 × 10 cm) loaf pan with parchment paper, leaving a 3-inch (8 cm) overhang on both sides. Preheat the oven to 325°F (160°C).

• Place the oats in the bowl of a food processor and pulse into a fine meal. Add the walnuts and pulse until very finely chopped. Add the cacao powder, coconut, flaxseed, salt, and cinnamon and pulse until just combined. Add the drained dates and almond butter and pulse a few times, until dispersed, then continue to pulse until the mixture is combined. Pulse in the almond or oat milk.

• Press the mixture firmly into the prepared loaf pan. Top with the cacao nibs. Cover the mixture with the overhanging parchment paper and refrigerate until set, about one hour. Remove from the pan by lifting the edges of the parchment paper. Cut into eighteen squares.

• Store bars in a sealed container in the refrigerator for up to one week, or in the freezer for three months.

MUESLI BOWLS

Sleep-inducing foods: almond, walnut, oat, sunflower seed, tart cherry, flaxseed, cacao, almond milk, dairy

YIELD: 6 SERVINGS

One of the best late-night snacks is a bowl of cereal, but all that extra sugar is bound to keep you awake. The alternative? Muesli. A blend of nuts, seeds, dried fruit, and cinnamon, this Swiss breakfast bowl is just as satisfying at the end of the day. Keep a jar of the dry mix in your fridge, and add yogurt or milk to serve. If you have fresh berries lying around, you're definitely going to want to mix in a few handfuls.

INGREDIENTS

¼ cup (38 g) raw almonds

¼ cup (30 g) raw walnuts

1 cup (90 g) rolled oats

¼ cup (35 g) toasted sunflower seeds

3 tablespoons dried tart cherries

3 pitted dates, finely chopped

2 tablespoons ground flaxseed

2 tablespoons cacao nibs

1 tablespoon chia seeds

½ teaspoon cinnamon

Pinch kosher salt

Almond milk, low-fat milk, or plain yogurt

DIRECTIONS

• Preheat the oven to 325°F (160°C). Spread the almond and walnuts on a sheet pan and toast for ten to fifteen minutes, tossing occasionally, until golden and fragrant. Set aside to cool. When cool, roughly chop the nuts.

• Combine the almonds and walnuts with remaining ingredients except for the milk in a bowl. Transfer to a jar with a lid and seal. When ready to serve, pour a heaping ⅓ cup (80 g) muesli into a bowl and cover with milk or yogurt.

• Store the remaining muesli in a sealed container in the refrigerator and use within three months.

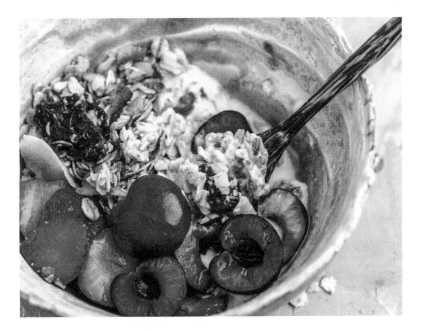

SINGLE-SERVING CACAO-CHUNK COOKIE

Sleep-inducing foods: flaxseed, almond butter, oat, cacao

YIELD: 1 COOKIE

Making a large batch of cookies is great fun, but sometimes all you need at the end of the day is one big cookie. This nutrient-dense, vegan, and gluten-free cookie is made with almond butter, maple syrup, and oat flour (though you can sub in regular or whole wheat if you're not gluten free!). The coolest part of making this dough is the flax egg. When you mix ground flaxseed with water, it forms a gel that binds dough together just like an egg.

INGREDIENTS

1 teaspoon ground flaxseed

1 tablespoon unsweetened almond butter

2 tablespoons maple syrup

½ teaspoon vanilla extract

3 tablespoons oat flour*

⅛ teaspoon baking powder

1 tablespoon bittersweet chocolate, roughly chopped

Flaky sea salt

*You can buy premade oat flour or grind 3 tablespoons rolled oats in the food processor. You can also substitute all-purpose or whole-wheat flour for the oat flour.

DIRECTIONS

• Preheat the oven to 350°F (175°C) and place a small piece of parchment paper on a sheet pan. Mix the flaxseed with 1 tablespoon water and let sit for five minutes.

• Whisk together the almond butter, maple syrup, vanilla extract, and flaxseed mixture in a medium bowl.

• Stir in the flour and baking powder until a dough forms, then add the chocolate.

• Shape the dough into a cookie about ½ inch (1 cm) thick. Top with a shower of flaky sea salt. Bake for ten minutes.

SWEET-AND-SALTY PEARS

Sleep-inducing foods: walnut, almond, pear, dairy

YIELD: 2 SERVINGS

Have you ever ended the night with an apple and peanut butter or cubed cheddar? This is like that but way more exciting, using pear wedges topped with toasted nuts, tangy chèvre, and a honey–olive oil dressing. This sort-of fruit salad is simple enough to throw together for yourself, yet at the same time looks festive enough to serve to late-night guests.

INGREDIENTS

2 tablespoons raw walnuts

2 tablespoons raw almonds

2 tablespoons honey

2 teaspoons extra-virgin olive oil

1 Bosc or Anjou pear, cut into
¼-inch-thick (6 mm) wedges

2 tablespoons chèvre, crumbled

Flaky sea salt

Freshly ground black pepper

DIRECTIONS

• Preheat the oven to 325°F (160°C). Spread the walnuts and almonds on a sheet pan and toast for ten to fifteen minutes, tossing occasionally, until golden and fragrant. Set aside to cool. Use a measuring cup or the bottom of a saucepan to gently crush the nuts.

• Whisk together the honey and olive oil.

• Transfer the pear slices onto a plate and top with the chèvre, crushed nuts, honey–olive oil mixture, flaky sea salt, and black pepper.

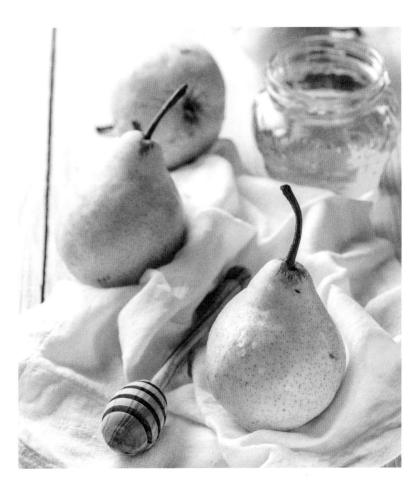

SMASHED-AVOCADO CRACKERS WITH SUNFLOWER CRUMBLE

Sleep-inducing foods: sunflower seed, avocado, whole wheat, tomato, dairy

YIELD: 2 SERVINGS

When you just can't wait until breakfast for avocado toast, make a few of these smashed-avocado crackers with sweet cherry tomatoes and salty feta. Though it may seem annoying to break out the food processor at the end of the night for seeds, the spiced sunflower–nutritional yeast crumble is hands down the best part of this snack.

INGREDIENTS

¼ cup (35 g) toasted sunflower seeds

2 teaspoons extra-virgin olive oil, plus more for drizzling

2 teaspoons nutritional yeast

¼ teaspoon cumin

¼ teaspoon kosher salt

1 avocado, halved and pitted

4 whole-wheat crackers

4 cherry tomatoes, thinly sliced

1 tablespoon feta, crumbled

Kosher salt

Freshly ground black pepper

DIRECTIONS

• Combine the sunflower seeds, olive oil, nutritional yeast, cumin, and salt in a food processor and pulse a few times until the seeds are broken up a bit.

• Spread a quarter of the avocado onto each cracker. Divide the sunflower crumble evenly among the crackers. Top each cracker with the tomato and feta, season with salt and black pepper, and drizzle with olive oil.

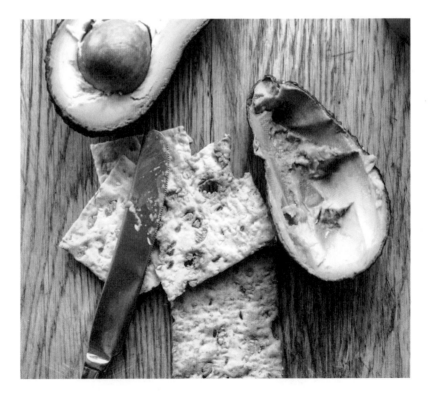

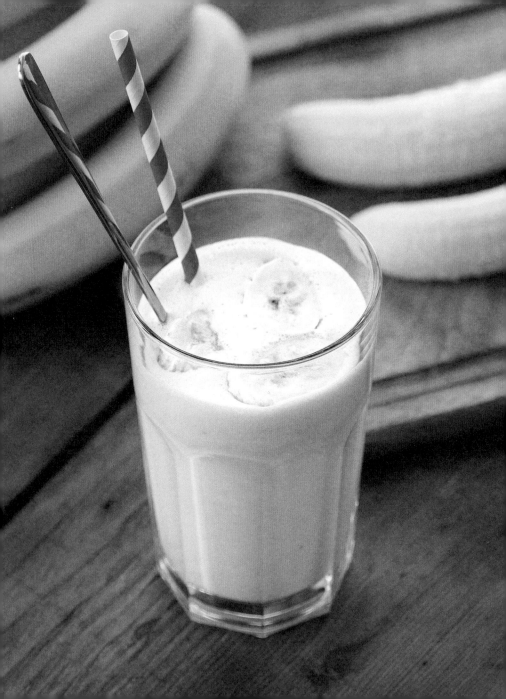

BANANA BREAD SMOOTHIE

Sleep-inducing foods: oat, banana, almond milk, walnut, cacao

YIELD: 1 SERVING

Basically a thick slice of banana bread in beverage form, this smoothie is a dream when you need something sweet on a warm evening. It's best to freeze individual slices of banana on a sheet pan, then pile them all into a plastic bag or container. Frozen food won't stick together in giant chunks that can wear out blender motors.

INGREDIENTS

2 tablespoons rolled oats

½ banana, frozen, roughly chopped

¼ cup (60 ml) almond milk

2 tablespoons chopped raw walnuts

½ teaspoon vanilla extract

2 teaspoons cacao nibs

Ice, optional

DIRECTIONS

• Combine all the ingredients in a high-power blender and blend until smooth. If it's proving difficult to blend, add in ¼ cup (60 ml) more almond milk. If you like thicker smoothies, blend in ice by the handful until you achieve the desired texture. Pour into a glass and drink immediately.

PEACHES-AND-CREAM SMOOTHIE

Sleep-inducing foods: peach, almond milk, dairy, flaxseed

YIELD: 1 SERVING

PSA: Baking peaches makes them taste even more peachy, even if you're not using super-seasonal, ripe fruit. (And yes, you can amplify the flavor of most other fruits the same way.) If it's the middle of winter, though, you might want to defrost and then bake frozen peach slices.

Provided you don't eat all of the jammy baked peaches straight from the sheet pan, they make a killer smoothie. Blend them up with yogurt and cinnamon for a drink that's basically a liquefied whipped cream–topped peach cobbler.

INGREDIENTS

1 large yellow peach, sliced

1 teaspoon honey

Pinch kosher salt

¼ cup (60 ml) almond milk

¼ cup (56 g) low-fat Greek yogurt

1 tablespoon ground flaxseed

¼ teaspoon cinnamon

DIRECTIONS

• Preheat the oven to 400°F (205°C). Toss the peach slices with honey and salt, and bake for ten minutes. Let cool.

• Combine the cooled peaches and remaining ingredients in a high-power blender and blend until smooth. Pour into a glass and drink immediately.

ICED MINTY PASSION FRUIT TEA

Sleep-inducing foods: peppermint tea, passion fruit tea

YIELD: 2 SERVINGS

This is the drink to brew when you're craving a tall glass of sweet tea at the end of the day but don't want the caffeine. If you like, brew an extra-large batch of tea at the beginning of the week, store it in the fridge, and have a glass whenever you need to wind down with a cool sipper.

INGREDIENTS

2 bags peppermint tea

2 bags passion fruit tea

½ lemon, juiced

2 tablespoons honey

Ice

DIRECTIONS

• Bring 4 cups (1 L) of water to a boil. Pour into a large liquid measuring cup or pitcher with the peppermint and passion fruit tea bags and steep for five minutes. Remove passion fruit tea bags and steep for another five minutes, then remove the peppermint tea bags. Transfer the mixture to the refrigerator and cool for at least two hours.

• After the mixture has cooled, stir in the lemon juice and honey. Serve in glasses over ice.

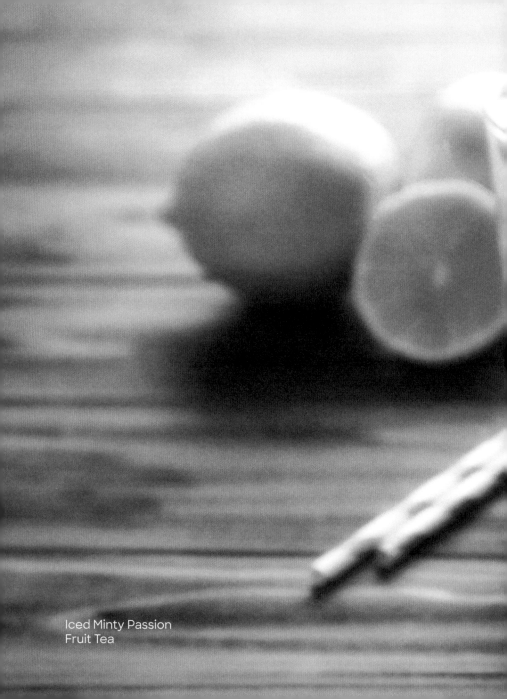

Iced Minty Passion
Fruit Tea

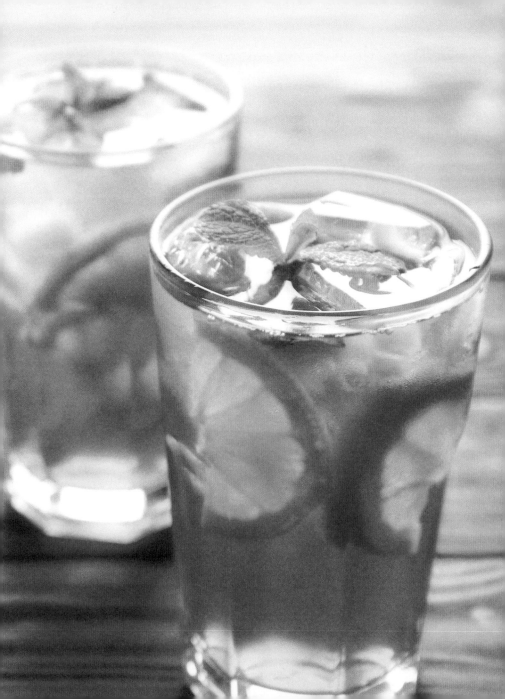

SPICED ALMOND MILK

Sleep-inducing food: almond milk

YIELD: 1 SERVING

Fun fact: When you blend almond butter with water, it instantly becomes a toasty almond milk—magic. Even better, if you mix that milk with warm spices like turmeric, cinnamon, ginger, and black pepper, you've got a sweet, subtly spicy drink you'll want to curl up with before getting ready for bed. This honey-sweetened milk is just as delightful warm as it is over ice.

INGREDIENTS

2 tablespoons unsweetened almond butter

¼ teaspoon turmeric

¼ teaspoon cinnamon

¼ teaspoon ground ginger

Freshly ground black pepper

1 teaspoon honey

DIRECTIONS

• Combine the almond butter, turmeric, cinnamon, ginger, and a pinch of black pepper in a high-power blender with 1 cup (240 ml) water. Blend until the mixture is smooth and frothy.

• For an iced drink, blend in honey, then serve in a glass over ice. For a hot drink, heat the mixture in a small saucepan over medium low heat until it simmers, let it cool slightly, then stir in honey. Pour into a mug and drink immediately.

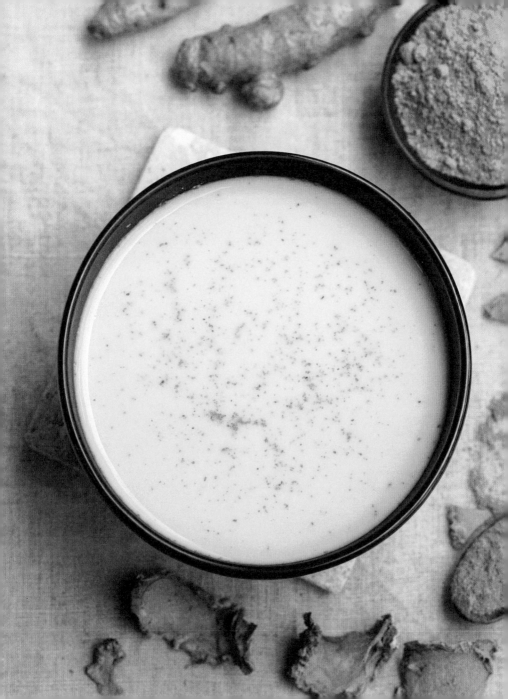

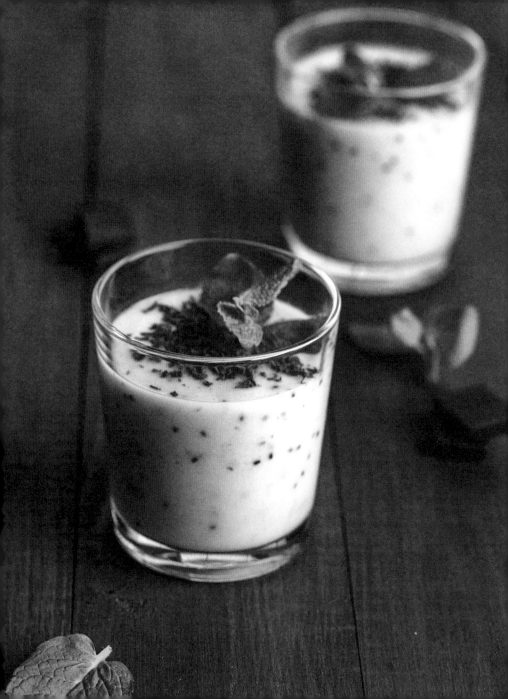

MINT-CACAO SHAKE

Sleep-inducing foods: almond/oat milk, leafy green, avocado, almond butter, dried fruit, cacao

YIELD: 1 SERVING

A mint–chocolate chip shake for bedtime, this date-sweetened smoothie is impossibly creamy thanks to half an avocado. Dye it bright green like the ice cream with a handful of spinach (and hey, bonus nutrients!), and let fresh mint and cacao nibs bring out a subtler version of the classic flavor. Use chopped dark chocolate in place of the nibs for a sweeter treat. A note on dates: If you can't find the smaller Deglet Noor dates, half a large Medjool date will work.

INGREDIENTS

½ cup (120 ml) almond or oat milk

¼ cup (39 g) frozen spinach

½ avocado

¼ cup (7 g) fresh mint

1 tablespoon unsweetened almond butter

1 pitted Deglet Noor date

Ice

2 tablespoons cacao nibs

DIRECTIONS

• Combine the milk, spinach, avocado, mint, almond butter, date, and a handful of ice in a high-power blender and blend until smooth.

• Stir in the cacao nibs. Pour into a glass and drink immediately.

LEMON-GINGER CHAMOMILE TEA

Sleep-inducing food: chamomile tea

YIELD: 2 SERVINGS

Feeling under the weather? This lemon-ginger drink will save you. With plenty of spicy, freshly grated ginger and soothing honey, this enhanced chamomile tea will have you ready to crawl into bed in no time. To really knock out any sickness from your system, double the ginger and grate a raw garlic clove into the brew.

INGREDIENTS

2 bags chamomile tea

1 teaspoon grated fresh ginger

1 lemon, zested and juiced

2 teaspoons honey

DIRECTIONS

• Bring 2 cups (470 ml) of water to a boil. Divide the water between two mugs, place 1 chamomile tea bag in each, and let steep for five minutes. Remove the tea bags and set the tea aside to cool slightly.

• In a small bowl, combine the ginger, lemon zest and juice, and honey. Stir half of the mixture into each mug. Drink immediately.

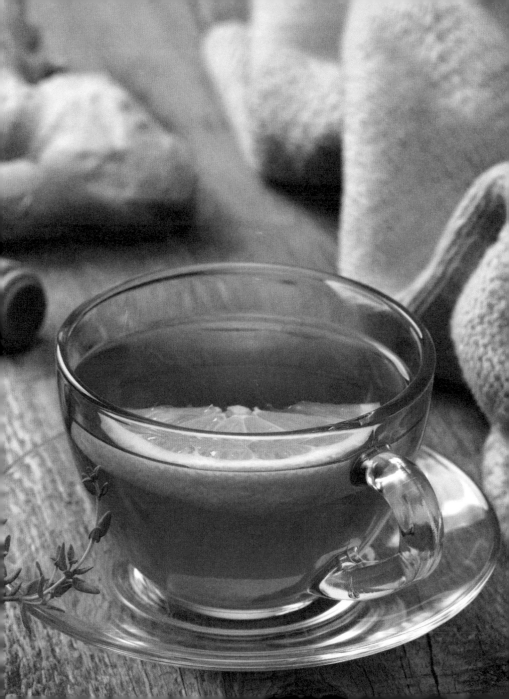

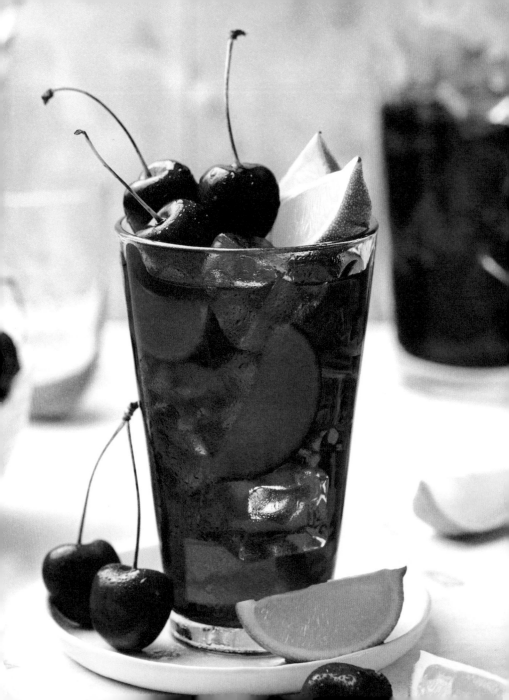

TART CHERRY-LIME SODA

Sleep-inducing food: tart cherry

YIELD: 1 SERVING, PLUS EXTRA CHERRY SYRUP

Most Italian sodas (fruit syrup and seltzer) you find at restaurants slant very sweet, but when you make your own syrup, the balance is just right. When making the syrup, choose an unsweetened tart-cherry juice with a short ingredients list. The best part is that this recipe makes plenty of extra-tart cherry-lime syrup, so you can have one of these bad boys every night.

INGREDIENTS

2 cups (470 ml) tart-cherry juice

¼ cup (32 g) granulated sugar

1 lime, zested and juiced

Ice

Seltzer

Lime wedges, for garnish

DIRECTIONS

• Combine the cherry juice, sugar, and lime zest and juice in a medium saucepan over medium heat. Bring the mixture to a boil, then lower the heat to simmer. Let the mixture thicken slightly, fifteen to twenty minutes. Pour the syrup into a glass jar or bottle and let it cool to room temperature.

• Pour 1 tablespoon of the syrup into a highball glass. Fill the glass with ice, then top with seltzer and a lime wedge. Drink immediately. Store extra syrup in an airtight container in the fridge for up to two weeks.

LAVENDER STEAMER

Sleep-inducing foods: oat/almond, dried fruit, lavender tea

YIELD: 1 SERVING

A latte without the coffee is the best thing to sip on at the end of the day. Start with date-sweetened milk (almond or oat will do nicely, though you can use regular milk here if you prefer), then gently heat the milk with lavender tea bags. For extra calming vibes, sip on this in the tub with lavender bath salts.

INGREDIENTS

1 cup (240 ml) unsweetened oat or almond milk

½ teaspoon vanilla extract

1 Deglet Noor date, pitted

2 bags lavender tea

DIRECTIONS

• Pour the milk into a high-power blender. Add the vanilla and date. Blend the mixture on high until smooth and frothy.

• In a small saucepan, combine the milk mixture and tea bags over medium low heat until it simmers. Let steep for ten minutes. Discard the tea bags. Pour into a mug and drink immediately.

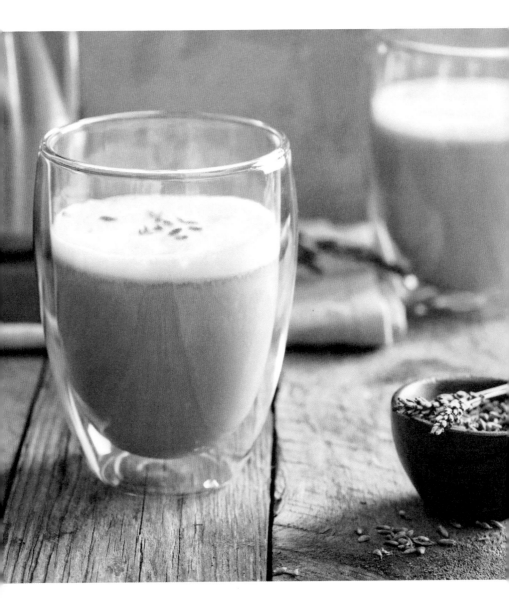

ORANGE TONIC

Sleep-inducing foods: chamomile tea, orange

YIELD: 2 SERVINGS

This drink may taste like rays of early morning sunshine, but it'll put you right to sleep. And while store-bought, unsweetened carrot juice works great here, make sure you squeeze your own oranges—there's just no comparison. For an extra-tart drink, make lemon ice cubes (go half water, half lemon juice) the night before.

INGREDIENTS

2 bags chamomile tea

2 oranges, juiced

¼ cup (60 ml) carrot juice

2 teaspoons grated fresh ginger

Ice

Seltzer

Lemon slices, for garnish

DIRECTIONS

• Bring ½ cup (120 ml) water to a boil. Pour into a large liquid measuring cup or pitcher with the chamomile tea bags and steep for five minutes. Remove the tea bags and let cool completely in the refrigerator, at least two hours.

• When the tea is cooled, whisk in the orange juice, carrot juice, and ginger.

• Fill two glasses with ice. Divide tea mixture between glasses and top with a float of seltzer. Garnish with lemon slices and drink immediately.

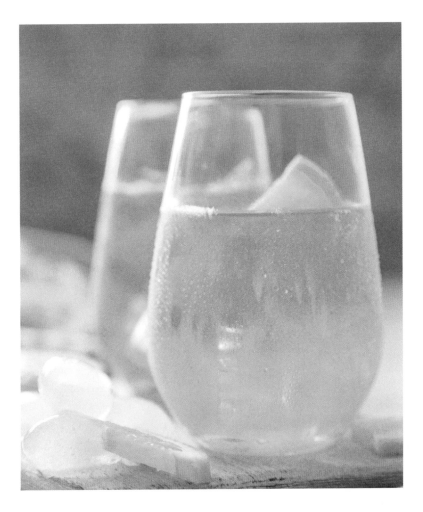

Glossary

adenosine: A chemical that plays a role in regulating the homeostatic system and helps promote sleep.

antioxidant: A substance that protects cells from damage caused by free radicals in the body.

blue light: The type of light emitted by electronic screens. This short-wavelength light looks like sunlight to our brains, making it particularly harmful to melatonin production. Studies have found it suppresses the release of melatonin by more than 50 percent.

chronotype: This term refers to whether you are a morning person (meaning you feel your best in the morning and go to sleep early) or an evening type (you tend to stay up later and perform better later in the day). Your chronotype is determined by your genes.

circadian system: One of two systems that regulates sleep. The circadian system works on an approximately twenty-four-hour rotation and responds to daylight and darkness in our environments. While circadian rhythms are naturally regulated within the body, external factors—sunlight specifically—also affect them.

free radicals: Unstable molecules in cells that can damage other molecules, such as DNA, and lead to disease.

ghrelin: The hormone that stokes our appetite, making us feel hungry.

homeostatic system: The second system that regulates sleep. It is a self-regulating system that helps keep your body stable and at optimal fitness for survival.

hygge: Pronounced *hoo-gah*, a Danish term which loosely translates to a "cozy way of life." This Nordic tradition is about getting back to basics, prioritizing what's important, and simplifying your life.

leptin: The hormone that signals us to stop eating, reducing our appetite.

meditation: Essentially, a state of stillness where no effort is necessary. Through that stillness, meditating helps you cultivate a deeper awareness of your body and mind. It helps you notice how your body feels and become aware of the passing thoughts and feelings in your mind.

melatonin: A sleep-inducing hormone naturally secreted by the pineal gland. When released into the bloodstream, it circulates throughout the body, where it binds to receptors found in the pituitary gland, ovaries (in women), blood vessels, and the intestinal tract. These receptors then signal to the body that it is time to sleep.

mind-body connection: The idea that the thoughts and beliefs in our minds can positively (or negatively!) influence our physical health.

non–rapid eye movement (NREM) sleep: NREM is the first cycle of sleep we go through. Also known as dreamless sleep, it consists of four stages, each of which lasts approximately five to fifteen minutes.

rapid eye movement (REM) sleep: REM sleep typically begins about ninety minutes after we fall asleep. This is the period of sleep when we dream, and it is characterized by certain physiological changes, including faster breathing, increased brain activity, rapid eye movement, and muscle relaxation. Our brains work to store, organize, and enhance memories and learning during this period.

self-care: A buzzword in the wellness world, self-care means shifting your mindset away from what you have to do—for your family, for work, for other people—and focusing on what you need in the moment.

sleep hygiene: The act of controlling your sleep behaviors and environments in an effort to optimize your sleep. It encompasses all the things that you can control to set yourself up for a successful night's sleep.

suprachiasmatic nucleus (SCN): Known as our "internal clock," the SCN is located in the hypothalamus in the brain. It is a small cone-shaped structure that controls many of the functions of the autonomic nervous system, including our circadian rhythms. It's the reason why you (should) feel sleepier at night and more awake during the day.

tryptophan: An essential dietary amino acid and a precursor to melatonin production. It's found in most protein-rich foods, especially chicken, turkey, eggs, cheese, fish, seeds, nuts, and legumes.

Bibliography

"2013 International Bedroom Poll: Summary of Findings." Accessed April 15, 2019. National Sleep Foundation. https://www .sleepfoundation.org/sites/default/ files/inline-files/RPT495a.pdf.

Alzoubi, Karem H., et al. "Chronic Melatonin Treatment Prevents Memory Impairment Induced by Chronic Sleep Deprivation." *Molecular Neurobiology* 53, no. 5 (July 2016): 3439–47. https://link .springer.com/article/10.1007/ s12035-015-9286-z.

"Antioxidants Explained in Human Terms." Healthline. https://www .healthline.com/nutrition/ antioxidants-explained#section1.

Asarnow, Lauren D., et al., "Evidence for a Possible Link between Bedtime and Change in Body Mass Index." *Sleep* 38, no. 10 (October 1, 2015): 1523–7. https://www.ncbi.nlm.nih .gov/pmc/articles/PMC4576325.

"Asleep on the Job: Causes and Consequences of Employees' Disrupted Sleep and How Employers Can Help." Virgin Pulse Institute. Accessed April 15, 2019. https:// connect.virginpulse.com/asleep-on -the-job-report-from-virgin-pulse.pdf.

"B Vitamins." MedlinePlus. Accessed June 23, 2019. https://medlineplus .gov/bvitamins.html.

BaHammam, Ahmed S., et al. "Distri- bution of Chronotypes in a Large Sample of Young Adult Saudis." *Annals of Saudi Medicine* 31, no. 2 (March–April 2011): 183–186. https://www.ncbi.nlm.nih.gov/pmc/ articles/PMC3102480.

Bandyopadhyay, D, et al. "Melatonin Protects Against Gastric Ulceration and Increases the Efficacy of Ranit- idine and Omeprazole in Reducing Gastric Damage." *Journal of Pineal Research* 33, no. 1 (August 2002): 1–7. https://www.ncbi.nlm.nih.gov/ pubmed/12121479.

Bellipanni, G. "Effects of Melatonin in Perimenopausal and Menopausal Women: A Randomized and Placebo Controlled Study." *Experimental Gerontology* 36, no. 2 (February 2001): 297–310. https://www.ncbi .nlm.nih.gov/pubmed/11226744.

Bent, Stephen. "Valerian for Sleep: A Systematic Review and Meta-Analysis." *The American Journal of Medicine* 119, no. 12 (December 2006): 1005–12. https://www.ncbi.nlm.nih.gov/ pubmed/17145239.

"Blue Light Has a Dark Side." Harvard Health Publishing. August 13, 2018. https://www.health. harvard.edu/staying-healthy/ blue-light-has-a-dark-side.

Breus, Michael. *Good Night: The Sleep Doctor's 4-Week Program to Better Sleep and Better Health*. New York: Dutton Adult, 2006.

———. "Understanding Melatonin: How Melatonin Can Help Sleep and Bio Time." The Sleep Doctor. June 6, 2017. https://thesleepdoctor. com/2017/06/06/understanding -melatonin-melatonin-can-help-sleep -bio-time.

"Caffeine and Sleep." The National Sleep Foundation. Accessed June 1, 2019. https://www.sleepfoundation .org/articles/caffeine-and-sleep.

"Candle Safety Rules." National Candle Association. Accessed June 2, 2019. http://candles.org/fire -safety-candles/candle-safety-rules.

Celinski, K, et al. "Melatonin or L-tryptophan Accelerates Healing of Gastroduodenal Ulcers in Patients Treated with Omeprazole." *Journal of Pineal Research* 50, no. 4 (May 2011): 389–94. https://www .ingentaconnect.com/content/mksg/ jpi/2011/00000050/00000004/ art00006.

Chang, Anne-Marie, et al. "Evening Use of Light-Emitting Ereaders Negatively Affects Sleep, Circadian Timing, and Next-Morning Alertness." *Proceedings of the National Academy of Sciences of the United States of America* 112, no. 4 (January 27, 2015): 1232–7. First published December 22, 2014. https://doi.org/10.1073/ pnas.1418490112.

Cherasse, Yoan, and Yoshihiro Urade. "Dietary Zinc Acts as a Sleep Modulator." *International Journal of Molecular Sciences* 18, no. 11 (November 2017): 2334. https:// www.ncbi.nlm.nih.gov/pmc/articles/ PMC5713303.

Cherry, Kendra. "9 Common Dreams and What They Supposedly Mean." Verywell Health. Accessed August 16, 2019. https://www.verywellmind.com/ understanding-your-dreams-2795935.

Corliss, Julie. "Mindfulness Meditation Helps Fight Insomnia, Improves Sleep." Harvard Health Publishing, Feb. 18, 2015. https://www.health .harvard.edu/blog/mindfulness -meditation-helps-fight-insomnia -improves-sleep-201502187726.

"Drowsy Driving: Asleep at the Wheel." Centers for Disease Control and Prevention. https://www.cdc.gov/ features/dsdrows driving/index.html.

Ferracioli-Oda, Eduardo, et al. "Meta-Analysis: Melatonin for the Treatment of Primary Sleep Disorders." *PLoS One* 8, no. 5 (2013): e63773. https://www.ncbi.nlm.nih.gov/pmc/articles/PMC3656905.

Gerritsen, Roderik and Guido Band. "Breath of Life: The Respiratory Vagal Stimulation Model of Contemplative Activity." *Frontiers in Human Neuroscience* 12 (2018): 397. https://www.ncbi.nlm.nih.gov/pmc/articles/PMC6189422.

Goel, Namni, Hyungsoo Kim, and Raymund P. Lao. "An Olfactory Stimulus Modifies Nighttime Sleep in Young Men and Women" *Chronobiology International* 22, no. 5: 889–904. https://www.tandfonline.com/doi/abs/10.1080/07420520500263276.

Gover, Tzivia. *The Mindful Way to a Good Night's Sleep*. New York: Storey Publishing, 2017.

Hammon, Claudia, and Gemma Lewis. "The Rest Test: Preliminary Findings from a Large-Scale International Survey on Rest." *The Restless Compendium: Interdisciplinary Investigations of Rest and Its Opposites*. Ed. Felicity Callard, Kimberley Staines, and James Wilkes. Basingstoke, UK: Palgrave Macmillan, 2016. https://www.ncbi.nlm.nih.gov/books/NBK453237/#ch8.s2.

Herxheimer, A., et al. "Melatonin for the Prevention and Treatment of Jet Lag." *Cochrane Database of Systematic Reviews* 2 (2002): CD001520. https://www.ncbi.nlm.nih.gov/pubmed/12076414.

"How Long to Wait Between Alcohol and Bedtime." Verywell Health. Accessed June 3, 2019. https://www.verywellhealth.com/wait-between-alcohol-sleep-3014979.

Hurtuk, A., et al. "Melatonin: Can I Stop the Ringing?" *Annals of Otology, Rhinology & Laryngology* 120, no. 7 (July 2011): 433–40. https://www.ncbi.nlm.nih.gov/pubmed/21859051.

Hussain, S. A., et al. "Adjuvant Use of Melatonin for Treatment of Fibromyalgia." *Journal of Pineal Research* 50, no. 3 (April 2011): 267–71. https://www.ncbi.nlm.nih.gov/pubmed/21158908.

"In U.S., 40% Get Less Than Recommended Amount of Sleep." Gallup. December 19, 2013. https://news.gallup.com/poll/166553/less-recommended-amount-sleep.aspx.

"Insomnia: Studies Suggest Calcium and Magnesium Effective." Medical News Today. Accessed June 3, 2019. https://www.medical newstoday.com/releases/163169.php.

"Insufficient Sleep Is a Public Health Epidemic." American Sleep Apnea Association. Accessed April 15, 2019. https://www.sleephealth.org/sleep-health/the-state-of-sleephealth-in-america.

"Is Melatonin a Helpful Sleep Aid—And What Should I Know about Melatonin Side Effects?" Mayo Clinic. October 10, 2017. https://www.mayoclinic.org/healthy-lifestyle/adult-health/expert-answers/melatonin-side-effects/faq-20057874.

Jacob, Stephanie. "The Truth about Beauty Sleep." WebMD. Accessed June 1, 2019. https://www.webmd.com/beauty/features/beauty-sleep#1.

Johansen, Signe. *How to Hygge: The Nordic Secrets to a Happy Life*. New York: St. Martin's Griffin, 2017.

Kohn, Linda, Janet M. Corrigan, and Molla S. Donaldson, eds. *To Err Is Human: Building a Safer Health System*. Washington, DC: National Academy Press, 2000. https://psnet.ahrq.gov/resources/resource/1579.

Konrad Kleszczynski and Tobias W. Fischer. "Melatonin and Human Skin Aging." *Dermatoendocrinology* 4, no. 3 (July 2012): 245–52. https://www.tandfonline.com/doi/full/10.4161/derm.22344.

Konturek, P. C., et al. "Role of Melatonin in Mucosal Gastroprotection against Aspirin-Induced Gastric Lesions in Humans." *Journal of Pineal Research* 48, no. 4 (May 2010): 318–23. https://www.ncbi.nlm.nih.gov/pubmed/20443220.

Li, Ya, et al. "Melatonin for the Prevention and Treatment of Cancer." *Oncotarget* 8, no. 24 (June 13, 2017): 39896–921. https://www.ncbi.nlm.nih.gov/pmc/articles/PMC5503661.

"Light, Sleep & School-Aged Children: A Complex Relationship." National Sleep Foundation. Accessed June 10, 2019. https://www.sleepfoundation.org/articles/light-sleep-school-aged-children-complex-relationship.

Long, Rujin, et al. "Therapeutic Role of Melatonin in Migraine Prophylaxis: A Systematic Review." *Medicine (Baltimore)* 98, no. 3(January 2019): e14099. https://www.ncbi.nlm.nih.gov/pmc/articles/PMC6370052.

Lyseng-Williamson, KA. "Melatonin Prolonged Release: In the Treatment of Insomnia in Patients Aged 55 Plus." *Drugs Aging*. November 2012; 29(11): 911–23. https://www.ncbi.nlm.nih.gov/pubmed/23044640.

Lundmark, P. O. "Role of Melatonin in the Eye and Ocular Dysfunctions." *Vis Neurosci.* 2006 November–December; 23(6): 853–62. https://www.ncbi.nlm.nih.gov/pubmed/17266777.

"Magnesium—How It Affects Your Sleep." The Sleep Doctor. November 20, 2017. https://thesleepdoctor.com/2017/11/20/magnesium-effects-sleep/.

Mao, Jun J., et al. "Long-term Chamomile (*Matricaria chamomilla L.*) Treatment for Generalized Anxiety Disorder: A Randomized Clinical Trial." *Phytomedicine* 23, no. 14 (December 15, 2016): 1735–42. https://www.ncbi.nlm.nih.gov/pmc/articles/PMC5646235.

Mass, James B. *Power Sleep.* New York: William Morrow, 1998.

"Meditation for Beginners." Headspace. Accessed April 15, 2019. https://www.headspace.com/meditation/meditation-for-beginners.

"Melatonin." Drugs.com. Updated May 20, 2019. Accessed July 9, 2019. https://www.drugs.com/melatonin.html.

"Melatonin." Encyclopedia Britannica. Accessed April 16, 2019. https://www.britannica.com/science/melatonin.

"Melatonin." FamilyDoctor.org. Accessed April 16, 2019. https://familydoctor.org/melatonin.

"Melatonin." Nicklaus Children's Hospital. Accessed April 16, 2019. https://www.nicklauschildrens.org/alternative-medicine/melatonin.aspx.

"Melatonin." Pharmacy2U. Accessed April 16, 2019. https://www.pharmacy2u.co.uk/melatonin.html.

"Melatonin and Sleep." National Sleep Foundation. Accessed April 16, 2019. https://www.sleepfoundation.org/articles/melatonin-and-sleep.

"Melatonin Content of Supplements Varies Widely, Study Finds." ScienceDaily. February 14, 2017. https://www.sciencedaily.com/releases/2017/02/170214162728.htm.

"Melatonin: In Depth." National Center for Complementary and Integrative Health. Accessed April 16, 2019. https://nccih.nih.gov/health/melatonin#hed3.

Moretti, R. M., et al. "Antiproliferative Action of Melatonin on Human Prostate Cancer LNCaP Cells." *Oncology Reports* 7, no. 2 (March–April 2000): 347–51. https://www.ncbi.nlm.nih.gov/pubmed/10671684.

Nagendra, Ravindra P., et al. "Meditation and Its Regulatory Role on Sleep." *Frontiers in Neurology.* April 18, 2012. https://doi.org/ 10.3389/fneur.2012.00054.

Ngan, A., Conduit, R. "A Double-Blind, Placebo-Controlled Investigation of the Effects of *Passiflora incarnata* (Passionflower) Herbal Tea on Subjective Sleep Quality." *Phytotherapy Research* 25, no. 8 (August 2011): 1153–9. https://www.ncbi .nlm.nih.gov/pubmed/21294203.

Pappas, Stephanie. "Why Do We Sleep?" July 2017. https://www. livescience.com/32469-why-do -we-sleep.html.

Peuhkuri, Katri, et al. "Dietary Factors and Fluctuating Levels of Melatonin." *Food & Nutrition Research* 56 (2012). DOI: 10.3402/ fnr.v56i0.17252. https://www .ncbi.nlm.nih.gov/pmc/articles/ PMC3402070.

"Research on Drowsy Driving." National Highway Traffic Safety Administration. Accessed April 20, 2019. https://one.nhtsa.gov/ Driving-Safety/Drowsy-Driving/ scope%E2%80%93of%E2%80%93 the%E2%80%93problem.

Rossignol, D. A. "Melatonin in Autism Spectrum Disorders: A Systematic Review and Meta-Analysis." *Developmental Medicine & Child Neurology* 53, no. 9 (September 2011): 783–92. https://www.ncbi .nlm.nih.gov/pubmed/21518346.

Scheer, F. A. "Daily Nighttime Melatonin Reduces Blood Pressure in male Patients with Essential Hypertension." *Hypertension* 43, no. 2 (February 2004): 192–7. https://www.ncbi.nlm.nih.gov/ pubmed/14732734.

"Sleep Basics." Cleveland Clinic. Accessed April 16, 2019. https:// my.clevelandclinic.org/health/ articles/12148-sleep-basics.

"Sleep Deprivation Described as a Serious Public Health Problem." American Association for the Advancement of Science. Accessed April 15, 2019. https://www.aaas .org/news/sleep-deprivation -described-seri ous-public-health -problem.

Stranges, Saverio. "Sleep Problems: An Emerging Global Epidemic? Findings from the INDEPTH WHO-SAGE Study among More Than 40,000 Older Adults from 8 Countries across Africa and Asia." *Sleep* 35, no. 8 (August 1, 2012): 1173–81. https://doi.org/10.5665/sleep.2012.

Taffinder, N. J., et al. "Effect of Sleep Deprivation on Surgeons' Dexterity on Laparoscopy Simulator." *The Lancet* 352, no. 9135 (October 1998): 1191. https://www.thelancet .com/journals/lancet/article/ PIIS0140-6736(98)00034-8/fulltext.

Tartakovsky, Margarita. "How to Analyze Your Dreams (and Why It's Important)." PsychCentral. Accessed August 16, 2019. https://psychcentral .com/lib/how-to-analyze-your -dreams-and-why-its-important.

Thompson, Jill. "How Ancient Humans Slept Before Electricity." Sleep Advisor. November 28, 2018. https://www.sleepadvisor.org /history-of-sleep/#Why_Ancient_ People_Engage_in_Biphasic_Sleep.

Tresguerres I. F., et al. "Melatonin Dietary Supplement as an Anti-Aging Therapy for Age-Related Bone Loss." *Rejuvenation Research* 17, no. 4 (August 2014): 341–6. https://www.ncbi.nlm.nih.gov/ pubmed/24617902.

"Understanding the Side Effects of Sleeping Pills." WebMD. https:// www.webmd.com/sleep-disorders/ guide/understanding-the-side -effects-of-sleeping-pills#1.

"Use of Complementary Health Approaches in the U.S." National Health Interview Survey (NHIS). https://nccih.nih.gov/research/ statistics/NHIS/2012/natural -products/melatonin.

Walker, Matthew. *Why We Sleep: Unlocking the Power of Sleep and Dreams.* New York: Scribner, 2017.

"What 'USP Verified' and Other Supplement Seals Mean." Consumer Reports. Accessed April 29, 2019. https://www.consumerreports .org/vitamins-supplements/what -usp-verified-and-other -supplement-seals-mean.

"What You Need to Know about Supplements and Drug Interactions." Consumer Reports. November 15, 2015. https://www.consumerreports .org/vitamins-supplements/ supplement-and-drug-interactions.

Whitbread, Daisy. "Top 10 Foods Highest in Tryptophan." My Food Data. April 10, 2019. https://www .myfooddata.com/articles/high -tryptophan-foods.php.

"Why Do We Sleep, Anyway?" Division of Sleep Medicine at Harvard Medical School. http:// healthysleep.med.harvard.edu/ healthy/matters/benefits-of-sleep/ why-do-we-sleep.

Winter, W. Chris, *The Sleep Solution: Why Your Sleep Is Broken and How to Fix It.* New York: Berkley, 2018.

Yi, C., et al. "Effects of Melatonin in Age-Related Macular Degeneration." *Annals of the New York Academy of Sciences* 1057 (December 2005):384–92. https://www.ncbi.nlm.nih.gov/pubmed/16399908.

Zhang, Lei, et al. "Melatonin Ameliorates Cognitive Impairment Induced by Sleep Deprivation in Rats: Role of Oxidative Stress, BDNF and CaMKII." *Behavioural Brain Research* 256 (November 2013): 72–81. https://www.sciencedirect.com/science/article/pii/S0166432813004634.

Zhou, J, et al. "Pink Noise: Effect on Complexity Synchronization of Brain Activity and Sleep Consolidation." *Journal of Theoretical Biology* 7, no. 306 (August 2012): 68–72. https://www.ncbi.nlm.nih.gov/pubmed/22726808.

Acknowledgments

I'd like to thank my editor at Sterling, Elysia Liang, for approaching me about writing this book, putting the wheels in motion, and helping me mold it into the gorgeous finished product you now hold in your hands.

I also must give a big shout-out to two renowned sleep specialists, Chris Winter, MD, (wahoowa!) and Michael Breus, PhD. Not only did they each write engaging, definitive books on the subject of sleep that helped me greatly in my research, but they also patiently walked me through the intricacies of melatonin and sleep via phone and email multiple times.

This book couldn't have happened without recipe creator extraordinaire Rebecca Firkser, who developed the incredibly delicious recipes in chapter 7. Additionally, I'd like to thank yoga instructor Ava Johanna, who created the soothing bedtime yoga routine you'll find in chapter 5.

Last but not least, I'm extremely grateful to my parents, Ellen and Michael. Thank you for being my constant support system in more ways than one, and for encouraging my writing career from the days of my handwritten short stories all the way to my first published book.

Picture Credits

Index

sources of, 20. *See also* Melatonin
supplements; Snacks for bedtime
tinnitus and, 27
tryptophan and, 20, 51, 53, 58, 86,
87, **133**
Melatonin supplements, 30–37
about: what they do for sleep, 30
before starting, things to know,
36–37
choosing/sourcing, 32–33, 37
for delayed sleep syndrome, 31, 33
dosages by condition used for, 33–34
for insomnia, 31, 33
for jet lag, 30–31, 33
for low melatonin production, 31
making, 33–34
medication interaction precautions,
35, 37
for menopause side effects, 31
reasons for using, 30–31
for short-term use, 31, 36
side effects possible, 34–35, 37
sleep hygiene and, 40. *See also* Sleep
hygiene
talking to doctor about, 36
timing doses, 37
Menopause side effects, 31
Mental games, pre-sleep, 65–67
Mental health, 6, 8–9
Migraines, melatonin and, 27
Mind-body connection, 73, **133**
Mind games, 65–67
Mint-Cacao Shake, *123*
Morning person, becoming, 82–83
Motivation, for improving sleep, 57
Muesli Bowls, *106–107*
Music, soothing, 67

N
Noise, for sleeping, 45
Non-REM (NREM) sleep, 16, **133**

O
Odors, sleep and, 48–49, 64–65
Orange Tonic, *130–131*

P
Pain, chronic, melatonin and, 27
Pajamas, sleep and, 47
Peaches-and-Cream Smoothie, *116*
Pets, sleep and, 47
Pineal gland, 15, 19, 22, 32
Plan for improving sleep. *See*
Five-week plan

R
Rainbow Fruit Salad, *90–91*
Rapid eye movement (REM) sleep,
16–17, 18, 42, **133**
Reading before bed, 67–68
Rest Test, 2
Rituals. *See* Bedtime rituals
Romesco Ricotta Toast, *88–89*
Routine, bedtime schedule, 72–73.
See also Bedtime rituals

S
Salted Honey Nut Chewy Granola Bars,
98–101
Scents, sleep and, 48–49
Schedule, sticking to, 72–73
Seasons, melatonin and, 22
Self-care, 56, **133**. *See also* Bedtime
rituals
Shades, blackout, 42–43

About the Author

Locke Hughes is a journalist, author, and health coach. Originally from Florida, she's based in New York City but escapes to the mountains of Park City, Utah, as often as possible. She graduated from the University of Virginia with honors in English and received a certificate in health coaching from Emory University.

Over her career, Locke has worked and written for a range of health and wellness publications, including NBC News, HuffPost, WebMD, *O, The Oprah Magazine, Greatist, Women's Health, Shape,* and *Self,* among others. When she's not sharing science-backed health advice, you'll find her in a hot yoga class, on a hike, or relaxing with a good book.